THE FIRST-TIME PARENT'S CHILDBIRTH HANDBOOK

THE FIRST-TIME PARENT'S

CHILDBIRTH HANDBOOK

A STEP-BY-STEP GUIDE
for Building
Your Birth Plan

Stephanie Mitchell, CNM, MSN, DNP

Illustrations by Amy Blackwell

ROCKRIDGE
PRESS

Series Designer: Julie Schrader
Interior and Cover Designer: Lisa Schreiber
Art Producer: Tom Hood
Editor: Kayla Park
Production Manager: Martin Worthington
Production Editor: Melissa Edeburn
Illustrations © Amy Blackwell, 2021.
Author photograph courtesy InFocus Photography by Jaren Turner. Makeup by Brittany Nicole of Pretty Please Beauty.

ISBN: Print 978-1-64876-200-0 | eBook 978-1-64739-584-1

RO

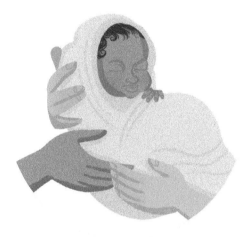

Contents

Introduction

For expectant parents, it's important to consider what they see as their main goals for labor and birth. In my experience, around the third trimester is when parents commit purposefully to planning, but the planning process can start at any time. Starting to ask questions earlier can lead to more informed decisions and a better chance for parents to reach their goals. Some clients start the process as soon as they receive a positive pregnancy test, others will start later, but the most successful and satisfactory birth experience is the result of purposeful planning.

Ainsley was among those who really hadn't put too much thought into the details of labor and birth. Her first and second trimesters had been complicated by an extreme form of nausea. Between the extra hospital visits and simply not feeling well, she hadn't really had time or energy to think about her plans for labor. At 28 weeks, what Ainsley knew was that she wanted to avoid a surgical birth at all costs. Over the course of the next several weeks, Ainsley was able to develop preferences and details specific for her labor, her birth, and the care of her newborn through childbirth education and discussion.

She presented her birth plan to the team when she arrived in active labor. The same plan followed her throughout different units of the hospital, and was incorporated into her specific plan of care with every shift change that brought in new care providers. For Ainsley, the written plan wasn't what was most important; she knew what her goals were. Instead, it was about the information she learned during the process of determining her preferences, and how this information allowed her to make knowledgeable and informed choices that specifically corresponded to her goals.

I ask my clients to consider the several stages, many details, and almost infinite options that influence their final birth route. Your birth will be unpredictable. Informed choices keep the unpredictability from becoming a hindrance to achieving your birth goals. No matter when you begin planning, your intentional preparation will allow you to be secure in your choices.

After caring for thousands of pregnant people and witnessing the transformation that happens through the process of developing and experiencing the unique labor and birth path, I am confident that purposeful efforts to learn and create an autonomous experience through the unpredictability of birth will result in a labor and birth experience you can reflect on proudly. By the time you complete this book, you will have a very important physical tool to assist you through the process of understanding your options, relaying your goals to your birth team, and accomplishing the labor you have prepared for.

A NOTE ON TERMINOLOGY

Language shapes our experiences and has the potential to cause harm to others when used incorrectly or without thinking through the implications. In acknowledgment of the diversity among maternal-child health professionals and those they work with, I aim to use gender-inclusive language.

I recognize that the term "maternal" may omit childbearing people who do not identify as mothers from the narrative, public health considerations, and data. We find ourselves in the midst of a system that continues to rely on this *maternal* term in larger public and international health spheres. It is important to me to be cognizant and vigilant about completely supporting both folks who identify as women and mothers and childbearing persons who do not but find themselves suffering under the same failed healthcare systems as others. This book uses gender-inclusive language to the extent possible.

When looking at data and information from the CDC or WHO, it's important to recognize the group that data and information seeks to protect and address. It is equally important to realize who may not be represented. I hold this tension throughout this book as I view health through a reproductive justice lens. When speaking in generalities, I attempt to use inclusive terms such as *childbearing people, pregnant people,* and *birthing people* to try to address systemic change necessary for all women, mothers, and childbearing people to thrive.

HOW TO USE THIS BOOK

Part One gives you the knowledge to feel comfortable and informed, because when you are provided more information about the topic, you can feel empowered to make the wisest decisions for your pregnancy. Use part one to lay a foundation for how the information you collect informs your decisions.

Part Two focuses on the aspects of labor and birth. We will start to construct your individualized birth plan as you continue to collect information and form preferences based on your goals. You will build on the foundations from part one and learn how to create a list of preferences. The birth plan template (see page 132) is a tool you can personalize to your unique needs. My hope is that you will use this book to define your own preferences, and that your birth plan will provide clear direction to anyone involved in your labor and birth.

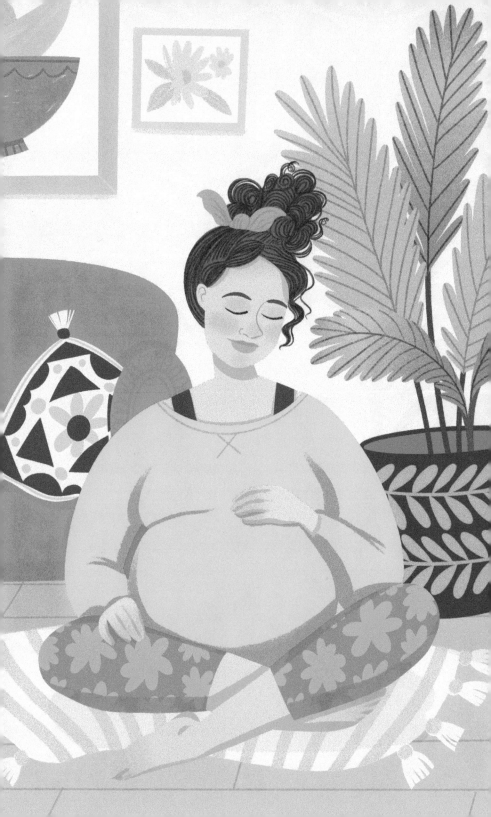

Keys for Success

This part of the book will help guide you through your birth preferences. You'll learn about mind and body goals as well as emotional labor. You'll see that the plan is the framework for effectively communicating and feeling secure in your choices. Key to the successful implementation of this plan is the information you build upon, which I like to think of as scaffolding, as you construct your initial birth plan framework. Exploring how your body and mind will feel most secure will be the basis for your more detailed decisions later.

Chapter 1

Mind and Body Basics

This chapter explores how the mind and body work together. This understanding will help you work toward your birth goals. After you have completed this chapter, you will begin to appreciate the ways you can physically prepare your body and your mind for labor, and for the minutes, days, and weeks after the birth of your baby. This physical and mental readiness will help you be well-equipped to carry out a successful plan.

BIRTH STORY: MIND OVER MATTER

Fear of the unknown is a barrier that people face in the weeks leading up to their labor, for fear often stems from a lack of information. Being fearful is not wrong or uncommon. The downside of going into a labor with unaddressed fear is that you can unintentionally become your own obstacle to achieving what you consider to be a successful implementation of your birth preferences. Common fears relate to pain, pushing, epidurals, tearing, or breastfeeding.

Carletta and Davina are two women who, though they did not know each other, shared a common fear. I met these women at very different times during their pregnancy journeys, and both were absolutely terrified at the idea of moving their bowels while pushing. Many people feel as though the pushing part of their labor feels like one long bowel movement, and it can be hard to differentiate between having a bowel movement and pushing. For Carletta, whom I cared for during pregnancy, we spent plenty of time discussing that if your bowel happens to be full, the baby will absolutely press down, upon exiting the vagina, on your lower bowels. If there is any stool in the lower rectum, the bowels will empty, at least in part. As we worked on her birth plan, the question emerged of what would happen if pushing led to more. Assurances were made that we would do what midwives have done for centuries: make an announcement to the room and hold a parade. Just kidding: I told her it is common practice for the midwives to discreetly remove any stool and continue to support the woman in labor. Part of the development of Carletta's birth preferences, then, related to handling hygiene issues because this issue was important to her.

I met Davina as she had just begun to push. With an epidural in place, she was surprised that the sensation of pushing felt like she was having a bowel movement, and she reacted by physically resisting. Davina's fear related to her interpretation of the sensation (having a huge bowel movement) versus what the sensation actually was (her baby's head pushing against her rectum from the inside), and this fear threatened to interfere with her pushing efforts. Davina shared the same fear as Carletta about having a bowel movement but was unable to address this fear before labor.

It's important to identify any fears you may have about the labor and birth process, so if you are unable to circumvent a situation, you have a contingency plan for how you would like things to be handled. Both Carletta and Davina went on to have normal vaginal deliveries with their dignity and pride intact. It's nice to know ahead of time some of the sensations to expect, so any fear won't get in the way of a productive birth experience.

Emotions

People who practice good mental health hygiene, such as using methods to mitigate stress and seeking access to mental health services, generally have a better time transitioning from their former roles as non-pregnant people into those of newly post-partum caregivers. The truth is that those with a history of pre-existing (diagnosed or undiagnosed) mental health disorders, particularly anxiety or depression, have a greater likelihood of developing an exacerbation of their symptoms in the postpartum period. To that end, pregnancy is the ideal time to check in with yourself to see how you have been feeling up to that point. Rapid physical changes and fluctuations of pregnancy-related hormones, combined with everyday stressors, can lead some women to disregard their mental health at a time when the emotional journey ahead requires as much close attention as their growing baby. The good news is that the upcoming section will cover basic mental health practices you can initiate at any point in your pregnancy to support the mental fortitude required throughout labor and during the immediate postpartum period. When you have a solid mental health plan in place prior to labor, as well as a plan for appropriate follow-up and aftercare, you should thrive both physically and mentally throughout your pregnancy and beyond.

MENTAL HEALTH TIPS

Your past responses to periods of stress can indicate how you might respond to the demands of pregnancy.

I recommend that you institute the tips throughout this section to support your mental health during every day of your pregnancy. Refer to these tips often to make sure you are not neglecting good mental health hygiene practices.

Touch base

Those who have had situational mental health concerns in the past should consider touching base with a licensed and qualified mental health care provider at least once during the pregnancy. Doing so will help establish care and create an anticipatory plan for support in the postpartum period.

Make time to be alone

Healthy ways to decompress during times of increased stress may include activities best accomplished intentionally alone. It is normal and healthy to want to decompress away from others. For those who may have limited means for alone time, take time to schedule a long shower or a soak in the tub to decompress privately.

Do a daily self-check-in

A self-check-in is asking yourself an intentional, black-and-white question every day of your pregnancy. Set an actual alarm for a time you are less likely to be inundated with other tasks. Remind yourself it is okay if some days are better than others. But the trick is this: Every day, routinely and predictably, set aside real time to ask about the person who is growing your baby safely inside of them. How are they doing today? (Pro tip: Do not have this conversation out loud or it could cause some concern to anyone overhearing you.)

Do what makes you feel good

One health benefit to indulging in pleasure is simply an increase in general satisfaction. Finding joy and indulging in it has many benefits. What makes you joyful? The list of infinite possibilities is too much for one numbered list. Take this moment to think about some reasonable things that absolutely, unequivocally make you happy. Be intentional about finding a way to enjoy them. Identify moments of happiness and joy, and allow yourself activities that make you smile. Do these things as frequently as you can throughout the entirety of your pregnancy.

KEY ADVICE: MENTAL HEALTH SELF-EXAM

Now that you have some simple self-check-in tools and understand the importance of daily practice, what do you do if you have not been able to decompress and are having some mental health concerns? The important thing to remember is you have identified your concern, and you should be proud you have been paying attention to the individual carrying your baby. As I mentioned, experiencing periods of feeling overwhelmed, emotionally drained, or even depressed throughout different points of your pregnancy is not uncommon. These emotions are normal. Sometimes, though, these normal emotions can become a more serious concern that should be addressed by a qualified professional.

Your provider will use specific questionnaires to help assess you for evidence of depression. However, being able to identify for yourself when you could use some mental health support is also helpful. Some questions to consider are:

- Do you feel like you are showing signs of depression, such as feeling sad, overwhelmed, or hopeless?
- Do you feel anxious or worried most of the time?
- Are you having feelings that interfere with your normal day-to-day functioning?
- Have you experienced panic attacks?
- Have you been blaming yourself more when things seem to be going wrong?
- Are you feeling sad, down, or miserable?
- Have you noticed that you have been crying more than usual because you are unhappy?

If you answered yes to any of these questions, it's time to talk to your provider about securing mental health support. If you are feeling helpless, hopeless, or in emotional pain to the point that the thought has crossed your mind to hurt yourself or others, tell your health care provider ASAP. This situation is considered a mental health emergency and should be treated in the same manner as any other emergency. Your provider will help create a plan to avoid physical harm.

Affirmations and Visualizations

Affirmations are generally any word or phrase that invokes a particular feeling, whereas visualizations are imagined scenarios that invoke the same feelings. In labor, helpful feelings are ones that call up safety, love, trust, and encouragement. To have the most impact, these affirmations should come from someone the person in labor trusts most. Like affirmations, visualizations will open up your mind to receive a message and emotion you are telling it to receive. The exercises below will guide you to listen to the person you should be trusting the most during this pregnancy. This person is who you are trusting to grow and nourish your baby and is the same person who, through their own might, will bring them earth side. You!

AFFIRMATIONS

Your brain believes what you tell it. Your brain is receiving hundreds of thousands of messages to which it sends corresponding actions to different parts of your body. Whether hunger or a warning, these signals are constantly talking to your body. By repeating positive affirmations to yourself, you are sending very powerful messages to your brain and body, which generally cooperate to obey your messages whether you say, read, or write them.

The following affirmations are examples you can draw from. Speak the messages you know to be true for you. Habits are formed over time, and affirmations work the same way. For best results, repeat them daily for 30 days.

+ My body is growing a strong and healthy baby.

+ I trust my body to tell me what it needs.

+ I trust my labor to start at its own perfect time.

+ I have the ability to accomplish anything I put my mind to.

+ My body is a capable and mighty vessel.

VISUALIZATIONS

Visualizations work best when you are in safe, quiet surroundings where you can sit or lie down comfortably. Practice initially for five minutes every day, but for gradually longer periods over time. Add more minutes each week so the brain has time to recognize the benefits and believe the visualizations. Start with the following visualizations to form a routine:

+ You are sitting comfortably on a grassy hilltop, perhaps on a blanket or with a pillow. In the far distance, you see the smallest dot on the horizon. Above is slight fluffy cloud cover, but the temperature is perfect, just how you like it. Allow your vision to focus on what is coming into focus: a large bird flying across the horizon. Watch the details of its graceful, slow glide across the sky. What do you feel? What do you hear?

✤ Imagine you are on the same hilltop, this time with your baby. Your baby has arrived safely. You are holding your baby. Feel the weight of your baby resting against your chest. Hear their soft breathing. What can you smell? What are they wearing? Feel how baby soft their skin is.

✤ See yourself sitting in a home familiar to you. Choose a space where you feel safe and comfortable. Imagine yourself walking into this room and sitting in a comfortable chair. Place your hands on your baby. What will you tell your baby about this space and why it makes you comfortable? Talk to your baby and describe in as much detail as possible the space around you. What will you tell them about how it feels, smells, and sounds?

Try to imagine these or similar scenes in as much detail as possible. Get creative. The goal is for you to find safe, calm spaces of retreat in your mind that translate to similar reactions in your body.

Breathing and Relaxation

In labor, you can't control contractions, but you can control your breathing. That's why breathing and relaxation exercises are helpful. Breathing patterns change as we accomplish certain tasks. Your brain connects slow, deep breathing to a relaxed and calm state. Alternatively, shallow breathing may signal stress to the body. These breathing techniques hold power to help you accomplish various tasks. You can train your breathing patterns to coincide with how you would like your body to respond. Like any new strategy, it takes practice to master the art of breathing

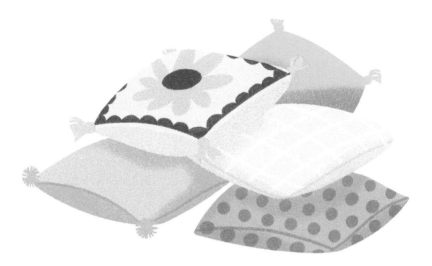

deliberately. Its mastery, though, will certainly help you through-out your labor and will assist you in accomplishing portions of your birth plan.

CALMING BREATH EXERCISE

Use this calm breathing exercise to de-stress and find comfort. Try several cycles of this exercise, paying attention only to your breath and how your body is moving with it.

Find a comfortable, quiet space in a seated position. Close your eyes to bring attention to your breath. After relaxing your body, take a slow deep inhale through your nose over the course of five seconds. Count for five seconds as you bring air in, and count again as you exhale. Over the course of the next several breaths, notice the rise of your chest as you inhale, the fall of your chest as you exhale. Next, over the same count of five, turn your head to the right, and as you exhale slowly, bring your head back to the center. Do the same thing on the other side, turning your head slowly to the left on your inhale, and back to the center as you exhale. It can be difficult for the brain to focus on doing two things at once, so moving your head while you breathe forces you to focus on both the movement and the breath, which removes other distractions.

ABDOMINAL BREATHING

When breathing is intentionally slowed and paced, this rhythmic breathing becomes the area of focus and diverts attention away from other areas of the body, providing maximum oxygen.

Lie on your back, putting a rolled towel or a pillow under one of your hips to displace your uterus off to one side (doing so prevents shortness of breath). Next, place one open hand on your abdomen and the other on your chest. As you inhale, pay attention to the rise of your abdomen. Focus on feeling the rise with each inhale and the dip with each exhale. Practice this for 10 breaths.

A Healthy Diet

Just as athletes prepare their bodies for physical tasks, pregnant individuals should emphasize good nutrition. Entering labor in a nutritionally depleted state can add an unnecessary layer of adversity as your body prepares to do the work required of labor and for the healing required postpartum. Whenever possible, swap processed food for fresh food. Instead of eating dried apple chips, choose an apple. Or instead of fruit cocktail, go for a fresh fruit salad. Fresh, whole, minimally processed food helps your body function at peak performance.

BERRIES

The antioxidants, fiber, and folate in berries are a few reasons you want to incorporate them into your pregnancy diet. Using the natural sweetness of fresh berries—added to whole grain cereals as a topping or incorporated into your favorite drink—is a way to avoid glucose dense sweeteners that can spike your blood sugar. Diets that incorporate berries have decreased risk of developing complications with blood pressure during pregnancy.

DATES

Dates assist with preventing anemia and regulating digestion, and they are packed with minerals that are good for your baby's bone development. According to one study, people who consumed five to six fresh dates per day during the last trimester of their pregnancy were more likely to go into their own spontaneous labor and less likely to need a medical induction.

DIGESTIVE DRINKS

A normal increase in hormones during pregnancy causes your digestion to slow down, which allows your body to absorb the maximum amount of vitamins and minerals from your digestive tract. Sometimes the digestion can be too slow and cause constipation. Drinks with such ingredients as apple cider vinegar, chamomile, coconut water, ginger, or nettle can assist with digestion, and beverages containing prunes or freshly squeezed vegetables may provide gentle relief from constipation.

ORGANIC, FREE-RANGE EGGS

Eggs are an excellent source of omega-3s and protein. The omega-3s help your baby's brain develop, and the protein acts as a building block of cellular growth. As a reminder, you are growing a lot of cells, and your body needs the protein. The dense protein is of huge benefit to your tissue strength, elasticity, and ability to repair itself when damaged.

ENZYME-RICH FOODS

Enzymes are nutrients that help with digestion. Remember Carletta and Davina (page 3)? When you have a normally functioning gut, your body is able to break down and digest all the good food you are putting into it, and your body is also in the optimal position to receive this nutrition.

GREEN VEGGIES

Leafy vegetables, such as kale, collard greens, and spinach, are building blocks for your red blood cells. They also contain the natural form of folate, known to prevent a particular defect in the spinal cord of developing babies.

LEGUMES

This group includes beans, lentils, peanuts, peas, and soybeans. Long after you have had your baby, these legumes will still provide you with essential fatty acids, fiber, and magnesium. Their wonderful fiber content helps prevent constipation and even hemorrhoids during pregnancy. Some legumes, such as chickpeas, are also thought to have additional benefits because of their essential amino acid composition, micronutrients, and phytochemical substances.

FISH

Fish, packed with important minerals, are a common source of omega-3s. Some types of fish cause concerns in pregnancy because of their potential mercury content. Bigeye tuna, mackerel, swordfish, and tilefish should be avoided. Catfish, pollack, salmon, or light canned tuna fish are safer. Keep in mind that you should consume only cooked small fish up to three times per week.

ROOT VEGETABLES

Hearty root vegetables can commonly be found in stews and soups, but also taste great roasted, baked, or even juiced. Beets, carrots, sweet potatoes, and every imaginable fall-colored turnip count as a root vegetable. Root vegetables are digestion aids jam-packed with essential vitamins, minerals, and antioxidants for you and your growing baby. When incorporated into a healthy diet, they can even stabilize blood glucose levels.

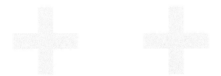

"WOMEN'S TEA"

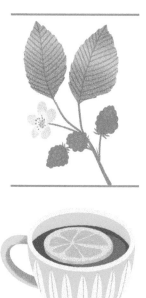

The chemical composition of red raspberry leaf tea supports a favorable uterine environment. This tea contains alkaloid fragine, thought to tone or prime the uterus to make it ready for labor. Your uterus must be able to produce strong and effective contractions so your cervix can open as your labor progresses.

You can find red raspberry leaf tea in your local grocery store. Loose tea leaves are best, but they can be a specialty item depending on where you live. Dried pre-packaged teas are a suitable alternative. Steep the raspberry leaf tea overnight for optimal benefits. Incorporate one to two cups daily from the second trimester and throughout pregnancy for the best results. Women who consumed red raspberry leaf tea throughout their pregnancy were found to have shorter labors, less preterm labor, fewer rates of induction, and less intervention.

Perhaps consider drinking tea as a ritual in which you incorporate other of your mental health hygiene practices and self-care rituals.

Getting in Shape

Healthy pregnant individuals should incorporate regular light exercise into their pregnancy routine. Returning to the athlete metaphor, your pregnancy can be looked at as several months of training leading up to one major exhibition. If exercise is not already part of your routine, pregnancy is the perfect time to start.

Incorporating regular activity will help with various aspects of labor and the postpartum process and may increase stamina, shorten the length of labor, and decrease your risk for postpartum depression.Whatever types of exercise you decide to implement, focus on intentional hydration before, during, and after your activities to prevent dehydration and overheating, which can be dangerous to you and your baby.

CARDIO

Regular cardio-oriented workouts have shown to be safe during pregnancy, but not without caveats. Pregnancy is not necessarily the time to implement a new physically intense cardio routine. A few low-impact exercises, such as swimming and walking, are more acceptable. These activities are good for increasing your heart rate, getting your blood pumping, and moving your muscles.

I've had patients become light-headed, get dizzy, and even pass out because they overextended themselves through vigorous exercise, despite being cautioned against it. Generally speaking, if you are not able to speak, your level of exercise is too intense for pregnancy. When you are short of breath, chances are you are also overheated, which should be avoided.

SWIMMING

Swimming is one of the best low-impact, high-cardio forms of exercise during pregnancy. Hormonal changes cause pregnant people to be more prone to strains and sprains, but because of the buoyancy afforded by water, this activity can give your joints a break. Not only does swimming tone your muscles, it also increases circulation and relieves the natural swelling that accompanies growing a baby. Swimming is also a natural method of using regulated breathing, which, as we discussed earlier, can be of major assistance when you are in labor.

WALKING

One of the easiest and safest activities for pregnant people is walking. A walking routine will build stamina, so you may find you are able to go for longer or more intense walks as the pregnancy progresses. You don't ever want to be out of breath or gasping for air when you are walking. It is okay, however, if you break a small sweat. The goal is to slightly increase your heart rate and build your stamina for physical activity. A fine goal is to connect a walking routine to an everyday event, like eating a meal. Incorporating a post-dinner walk will aid in digestion, expend energy, and prepare for the wind-down of the evening.

YOGA

Activities that increase flexibility, endurance, and strength will serve you well as you prepare your body for labor. Yoga accomplishes all these goals. If you are taking a yoga class not specifically designed for pregnant people, advise your instructor that you are pregnant and avoid hot yoga. Individuals who routinely practice yoga throughout their pregnancy find they have learned better breathing, relaxation, balance, plasticity, and overall improvement in self-efficacy and well-being.

Chapter 2

Labor and Delivery Basics

This chapter details what occurs during child-birth and provides insight on various induction techniques and interventions. You'll learn about the signs of labor and how to distinguish when active labor occurs. You will also learn about the stages of labor and some common reasons a birth may segue from the traditional and expected course. This chapter delves into how to engage your provider and birth team in conversations about your options. Whatever you decide, being prepared for all the various ways your particular labor can unfold makes going into your labor and birth space as smooth as possible.

BIRTH STORY: LABOR OF LOVE

The laboring process can be a quick or meandering experience or have an unexpected outcome. In the event that labor lasts more than 24 hours, rest assured you will see your bundle of joy soon. For Edith, labor started unexpectedly, and she found herself focusing on "when is soon?"

During her regularly scheduled 10 a.m. prenatal appointment a little after 40 weeks, Edith disclosed that she had been awake since 3 a.m. with what she thought might be irregular contractions. We were both surprised to find that her cervix was 6 centimeters dilated and 80 percent effaced, or thinned out. We decided she would return home to continue to labor until her contractions became more regular before heading to the hospital. I like to remind clients that it is impossible to nail down exactly when they will deliver their baby, even when we think we have an idea. Knowing I would be on call at the hospital that evening, my midwife brain was thinking, "She'll probably be at the hospital soon." But soon never came. Edith grew more nervous as the day progressed without regular contractions.

It wasn't until 6:55 a.m. the next day that I received one of my favorite pages: "Dr. Mitchell, please come to the Emergency Room for a midwife patient who feels like she has to push." When I saw Edith, I beamed from ear to ear. Edith visibly relaxed when she recognized a familiar face in the new environment. I didn't need to lay a finger on her to know she was about to have her baby, and Edith finally knew what *soon* meant as she began to crown. Within moments of my donning gloves, and after a few very strong purposeful and powerful pushes, Edith was skin to skin in the Emergency Department with her baby boy! Edith accomplished the birth that felt right for her. There was nothing that could have prepared her for such a long labor.

Her labor and birth story spanned the course of a day and a night, concluding a whole day later than everyone predicted. Her labor was long, but it was a labor of love, because she relinquished the idea of having to predict when it would conclude. She let her body create the birth story that was going to be her very own.

In Edith's case, labor came as a surprise when she found out she was 6 centimeters dilated. It came to a fierce, powerful, and surprising end when she delivered right as she arrived at the hospital. Your individual labor story is yours, however it unfolds. With certainty, it will be a labor of love.

Signs of Labor

Labor is not a lightbulb switch that flips on, but a process that shows itself through symptoms. Your body, even weeks before the actual start of labor, will start to exhibit some noticeable signs of the process, such as increased vaginal pressure, an increasingly regular pattern of contractions, loss of the mucus plug, or perhaps some spotting. You may perceive all these changes, some of them, or none at all. These changes can continue even up to the hours before active labor begins.

WITHIN WEEKS OF THE DUE DATE

Baby "drops"

Anywhere from days to weeks before labor, some people feel their baby a little lower in their abdomen than before. This shift means that your baby has descended into the very first position they will be in when you start labor.

Cervix dilates, effaces, and softens

As you go into labor, the cervix gets shorter and shorter as the opening gets wider and wider. It continues to stretch and thin out throughout labor until it is as thin as a piece of paper with an opening about 10 centimeters wide.

Cramps, back pain, and practice contractions

Some people find that in the days leading up to labor they have increased episodes of cramps and back pain, but early labor commonly consists of some form of cramping or back pain as well.

WITHIN DAYS OR HOURS OF LABOR

Mucus plug

The cervical opening is covered and slightly filled on one end with a jelly-like thick mucus that serves as a protective substance, or a cap to the entryway into the uterus. Losing the mucus plug in whole or in part cannot predict the start of labor.

Contractions

Where in your body you most feel contractions and how you describe their intensity also varies from person to person. Some people can expect to experience periods of contractions that last for a few hours, but with relieving measures, they eventually go away. When contractions indicate labor, they typically won't stop until you have had your baby.

A small percent of people will experience their water breaking before they go into labor. For others, this step may happen during active labor, and for some, not until right at the very birth of their baby. In most instances when your water breaks before labor, we expect that labor will start on its own within the next day.

The First Stage of Labor

You will experience three phases of labor. The first, early labor, is usually the longest portion for the first-time laborer. The phases of labor can be very obvious or subtle. Although the duration and intensity of each phase will vary from person to person, in every single normal labor and birth, all stages of labor will occur.

EARLY LABOR

Any combination of the "signs of labor" experienced over the past several days or even weeks will begin to increase in duration, intensity, and frequency. Contractions and the irregularity of your symptoms are the best indicator of early labor. During this time, the signs of early labor are tied to the effacement, dilation, and shortening of the cervix. Cervical dilation during this phase of labor will be 4 to 5 centimeters or less, and contractions can be anywhere from 5 to 20 minutes apart with a variable pattern. The goals of early labor are rest, hydration, nourishment, and continuous emotional support. A common complication of early labor occurs when people are unable to meet these goals. Interventions to help support these goals should be considered.

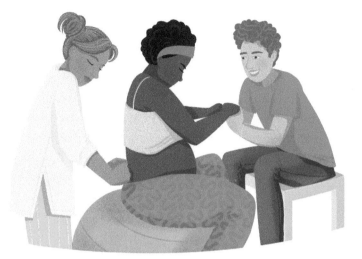

ACTIVE LABOR

During this time, one can expect that the regularity of contractions develops into a more predictable pattern of three to five minutes apart. As you transition into active labor, vaginal discharge increases, and the cervix is now focused on dilation, or opening. As active labor continues, it will become increasingly hard to sit still through contractions. Coping strategies and repetitive activities such as swaying, controlled breathing methods, or meditation can be used. Active labor typically lasts for a shorter amount of time than early labor, but the contraction pain of active labor is not as variable and usually remains just as intense and predictable throughout this phase.

TRANSITION TO SECOND STAGE

As active labor continues, it will become increasingly hard for the laboring person to sit still through contractions. As labor shifts from its early stages into the active stage, the contractions will command the person's full attention. This phase is when people need to fully shift in how intentionally they use their labor support tools and other support mechanisms to cope with the increased frequency, duration, and consistency of contractions.

KEY ADVICE: INTERVENTIONS DURING STAGE ONE

The objectives of all stages of labor are rest, hydration, nutrition, and emotional support. When people need help meeting their physical or emotional objectives because of protracted labor, fatigue, or inability to manage or tolerate contractions, interventions may be offered. Interventions can help one manage and tolerate symptoms as the labor continues. Other interventions are policy driven and will vary depending on your chosen birth space. Some interventions that can occur in the hospital are continuous external fetal monitoring, IV hydration, and both pharmacologic and non-pharmacologic methods to manage pain, ease nausea, or promote rest as your body continues to work. In all birth spaces, interventions can be both pharmacologic or non-pharmacologic with the same goals.

An ideal time to arrive at your birth space is in active labor, or sooner if you are unable to tolerate or manage your contractions from home. All birth setting interventions that assist people in meeting their early labor objectives will generally remain available to use throughout the entirety of labor. Interventions for pain control or symptom management should be led by the person in labor. The goal is to labor until you no longer want to labor without interventions. Interventions should be thought of as a supplement to assist the laboring individual. It's a good idea to know what interventions are available and used in your chosen birth space.

The Second Stage of Labor

Just prior to the cervix being completely effaced and dilated, the person in labor experiences a marked increase in contraction intensity. This moment delineates the end of the transitional phase and beginning of the second stage. The duration and frequency of contractions will likely stay the same, varying from two to five minutes apart, although some people experience a slight decrease in frequency. Your baby's head now has the job of navigating under the lowest arch of the pelvic bone through specific cardinal movements of their head as they traverse the nuances of your pelvis. As the uterus contracts, the baby's head presses down, which can cause the feeling of a full rectum (remember our friends Carletta and Davina?). The sensation of needing to empty the rectum will come and go, mirroring the timing of your contractions. In unmedicated labor, the sensation of increasing vaginal or rectal fullness eventually will result in some form of spontaneous bearing efforts. In this case, pushing throughout each contraction is led by the birthing person's intuition to push in the position for a duration and with the intensity that feels best.

For those experiencing labor with the use of interventions such as an epidural, there may be decreased ability to perceive vaginal and rectal pressure. In this case, your provider may rely on information from electronic fetal monitoring or a cervical exam to assess whether the second stage has begun. Your birth team can help coordinate bearing efforts with contractions to assist with the loss of sensation that comes with the epidural.

With or without intervention, the goals of the second stage should continue to be supported and encouraged by the people you have chosen to be with you in your labor space. For this reason, some people decide to hire a doula, a designated individual specifically trained in non-medical one-on-one labor support, to assist them throughout the duration of their labor and birth. At any birth setting, you can expect a provider and one to two trained assistants to be present. In hospitals, the trained individuals are typically nurses, and outside the hospital, you may be working with a nurse, a birth assistant, a second midwife, or an apprentice. The policies and practices of your chosen birth space may dictate who is essential to have at your birth and may also set parameters for people you may invite into the space.

The end of the second stage is memorialized by the specific date and time your baby emerges from your body, and at long last, when your labor contractions completely cease. Optimally, your baby is placed directly skin to skin on your abdomen or chest. This important time immediately following your baby's birth has been referred to as the *golden hour* because no interventions are critical enough to interfere with it. You can wait to weigh and measure the baby, administer medications, and even cut the umbilical cord while you bond and determine whether your baby is showing signs of wanting to feed.

KEY ADVICE: INTERVENTIONS DURING STAGE TWO

Uncommonly, interventions are used during the second stage of labor to help guide the birth of your baby's head under the pelvic arch, through the vaginal canal, and to the outermost part of your body, the perineum. These interventions are forceps, vacuums, episiotomies, and surgical births. Surgical interventions and the use of assistive instruments and procedures are not commonly considered an emergency, but some are counseled as urgent, leaving you a limited amount of time to consent. Not all interventions will be available at all birth places. Chapter 5 provides greater detail on interventions.

The Third Stage of Labor

The third stage of labor starts once your baby has been born and continues throughout the golden hour. The third stage will continue until you have successfully delivered your placenta. A typical third stage is expected to occur within 30 minutes of birth. Unmedicated birthers may experience an increase in cramping and bleeding, along with a build-up of vaginal or rectal pressure. These signs signify that the placenta has returned all of your baby's available blood back into your baby's circulation through the umbilical cord, and that the placenta has detached from the uterus wall, has passed through the cervix, and is in the vagina ready to be expelled. Pushing out the placenta requires minimal effort when compared to pushing out your baby because the placenta is a soft, pliable organ with no bones.

In cases where the placenta is delayed beyond a typical time-frame, breast- or chest-feeding is an intervention that releases a hormonal cascade of oxytocin, which causes the contraction of the uterus to assist in the expulsion of the placenta. During the expulsion, the uterus will continue to contract and immediately begin the work of returning to its pre-pregnant size. Contracting of the uterus after birth is also a protective mechanism to prevent excessive bleeding.

The conclusion of the third stage marks a time when some decide to cut the cord because the baby is finally separated from their previously life-sustaining organ. Some will choose not to perform intentional separation of the placenta from the umbilical cord and baby, instead opting to allow the cord to detach from the placenta on its own over the course of the next 3 to 10 days. Other options for the placenta include discarding it, donating it to research, burying it, or finding ways to memorialize this incredible temporary organ through jewelry or artwork. Some families make arrangements to ingest the placenta at a later date by converting it into pills, tinctures, or powders for use in the postpartum period, citing postpartum benefits or rituals that require use of the placenta. Your chosen birth space may have policies directing local regulations and guidelines for the proper use and storge of what is now legally considered medical waste.

Why Has My Labor Stalled?

Sometimes during the second stage of labor, we might observe a delay in the progression of dilation. When delays are identified, corrective measures can be employed, along with education and an exercise in patience, to bypass this common labor obstruction. A delay in labor progression can frequently be attributed to physical causes, emotional causes, and baby-related causes. When these causes are rectified, we see labor resuming in a more typical progression, resulting in a vaginal birth. In even the most concerted efforts, there will still remain a small number of labors that simply cease making cervical change beyond a certain dilation. On these occasions, when labor has completely stopped, one will need to consider a surgical birth.

PHYSICAL CAUSES

Recall that throughout labor, it's important to meet your basic human needs for nourishment, hydration, and emotional support. Recall also that as you enter into a more active labor, it may take more concentration and special focus on working through each contraction. It might not be uncommon to forget to take a sip of water after a contraction that required a fair amount of breathing exercises to work through. Basic human needs and normal physical functions do not cease just because you are in labor. For this reason, one-on-one labor support is critical to help you continuously address your physical needs. Activities such as routinely emptying your bladder, changing positon, eating, and moving around are all normal physical responses to help cope with labor. For those using an epidural, the loss of sensation and awareness of the lower half of the body will cause reliance on the labor support team to help you complete normal physical functions such as changing positions and emptying your bladder. The policy of your chosen birth space will dictate recommendations for interventions and restrictions of these normal functions. Allowing the body to address its physical needs, even when you need assistance, will help facilitate a normal progression of labor.

EMOTIONAL CAUSES

Anxiety about labor and birth are quite common. These emotions can be rooted in things you were told about labor, or might be related to fear of losing control or being physically exposed. The reality is some of these fears will go on to represent emotional stumbling blocks that can prevent the body from responding with typical progression in labor. Often, fear is rooted in lack of knowledge. Lean into the root of the anxiety, or how it developed. Identifying fear is the only way to traverse labor while allowing your body to focus on its physical and emotional demands.

Labor is a vulnerable state. During the most intense periods of labor, your brain will only be able to focus on one element at a time. Freeing space in your brain by removing the burdensome element of fear is not just some hippie midwife logic. The work of deconstructing fearful thoughts and making accommodations to assuage your fears prior to entering your birth space will persuade your body and mind to respond to the normal, expected work of labor without being overburdened by other heavy emotional work.

BABY-RELATED CAUSES

The position of your baby's head in relation to your pelvic bones may stall labor. The head can come out facing almost any direction, but the easiest passage is when the oval of your baby's head lines up with the ovals of your pelvic bones. This facedown position makes for a shorter and more even navigation of your passenger through the cervix as your labor progresses. In normal active labor, rhythmic movements during contractions, such as walking, squatting, lunging, leaning, pelvic rocking, or bouncing on a birth ball, can become instinctual if a person is allowed to labor uninterrupted. These movements encourage the baby's descent through the path of least resistance. Other times, the ovals don't line up in the path of least resistance, sometimes causing the passageway through the pelvic bones to take a little longer.

With the use of epidural anesthesia, movements are stunted or eliminated. With positioning aids such as a peanut ball or squatting bar, in addition to assistance with frequent position changes, your labor support person can help your body mimic normal body movements, thus assisting with alignment of the ovals of the head and the pelvis. When the cervix is stuck, changing positions regularly can help a baby achieve alignments of the ovals into the optimal facedown position, resulting in progressing cervical dilation.

KEY ADVICE: INTERVENTIONS AND BONDING AFTER BIRTH

As the baby regulates their breathing, they take in all the familiar sounds they've become accustomed to hearing—your beating heart, your voice, and the rhythm of your breathing. The birthing team may choose this time to administer two common interventions for newborns: vitamin K and eye ointment. Erythormycin, an antibiotic, is used as a precautionary measure to prevent an easily missed serious eye infection that in babies can lead to blindness. It is perfectly reasonable to delay the administration of this medication until after the first hour. Some people may choose to defer use of the medication altogether. Regardless of your plans for this medication, understanding the rationale and options are important when you're choosing whether to administer erythromycin as recorded in your written instructions.

When infants are born, they have a material in their blood that helps them create blood clots. This material develops over the course of several weeks. Until a good feeding routine is established, the levels of this clotting factor are low enough that if there were some covert bleeding in the infant, a rare but life-threatening condition could occur. The administration of vitamin K helps this blood clotting factor develop. Regardless of your birth space, you will have to decide whether to have this medication administered as a one-time injection or orally over the course of several weeks. You will clearly indicate these preferences on your birth plan.

Your chosen birth space may have some recommendations and policies in place about how you recover, as well as recommendations for timing and methods of administration of these medications. What does not change is your preferences for when, how, and along what timeline (if any) you would like these medications to be administered. While you are in the very earliest phases of your postpartum recovery, one of the jobs of the designated labor support person is to be sure your birth plan is readily available and accessible to those who need it. Your attention at this point will be exclusively on getting to know your new human—taking in every detail, including scents, feelings, and emotions while you are skin to skin. This time is not for the deliberation of non-emergency medication administration.

Uninterrupted bonding time is also an important step for newborns. Separation of the baby from birther by another individual should occur only if the situation is urgent. In some instances, a situation may occur in which an infant may need assistance transitioning to the outside world and with taking their first few breaths. If this happens, the disruption in bonding or the separation should cease as soon as the urgency resolves and the baby has resumed normal transition unassisted.

Chapter 3

Birth Plan Basics

This chapter will familiarize you with different components of your labor and birth and will help you formulate decisions that you will be called to make after delivery. Some of these decisions should be made well ahead of time. The key is to do your due diligence beforehand, reviewing the choices most in line with what you envision for your labor and birth. By doing so, any decisions made postpartum will be done with a general understanding.

BIRTH STORY: AN OUNCE OF PREPARATION

It is never too early to start thinking about the elements of your birth plan. You can make some basic decisions early on, whereas you may not be able to make others until you have more information. As always, flexibility is key. Evelyn is a client who used midwifery care for the duration of her pregnancy. She started working on her birth plan around 28 weeks, focusing on areas that were easy decision points. Strongly driven by her desire to have a low intervention labor and birth, she had settled into the thought of having a non-medicated labor.

As she delved deeper into the development of her birth plan, and started attending childbirth education classes, she realized she could make some important decisions at that moment, while other preferences developed as her pregnancy did. Needing the extra support for a non-medicated labor and birth, she decided to expand her labor team to include a doula for one-on-one labor support along with her partner and mother. The onset of the COVID-19 pandemic introduced further uncertainty to her plans. Hospital infection control restrictions limited Evelyn to one support person in labor. Remaining firm in her decision for a low-intervention, non-medicated labor and birth, as well as a desire to be accompanied by her chosen support team, she decided to look into an alternative birth space that would allow her full birth team to be present.

For Evelyn, having her full support team with her overrode the importance of her initial plan of a low-intervention labor and birth happening at a hospital with a midwife. At 32 weeks, Evelyn was transferred to a midwifery home birth practice to continue her care. She delivered non-medicated, at home, surrounded by her chosen birth team and the support and care of a homebirth midwife. Evelyn never could have predicted that she would have to modify one of her concrete decisions at 28 weeks. She prepared for the type of support she knew would be important to her, though, and that preparation helped her stay flexible and attain her goals.

A Two-Part Plan

Any successful birth plan will consist of two fundamental parts: the discussion plan and the birth plan. Using a two-part planning method will not only help you assert your boundaries during labor and birth, but also help you visualize the birth you want. This method will also let the birth team know how you want to use your birth plan as a tool to achieve your desired outcomes.

DISCUSSION PLAN

The discussion plan is just what you think it is—a piece of paper that is the vehicle of communication you take with you to your prenatal visits (unless you plan on memorizing all the options). The discussion plan will help you talk through labor options with your provider based on your interests. Think of the discussion plan as the tool you will use to gather pieces of information you need to make the most informed and personalized decisions for labor, birth, and beyond. The discussion plan IS your birth plan. It's part one of a two-part plan and, as such, is the very first draft you take with you to your prenatal visits so you can discuss various possibilities with your provider.

Goals and preferences for labor and birth go beyond the common expectation for a healthy outcome for you and your baby. The aspects of how you get to these outcomes are discussion points to have along the way and will vary from person to person. Those who do not express any preferences will get the standard hospital or birth center experience based on the experience, comfort, and preferences of the provider or birth space, and not on points important to the individual.

The discussion plan should include decisions you feel are nonnegotiable, along with decisions with plenty of latitude. Even if your plan is to follow every suggestion provided to you in your chosen birth space, the discussion plan will guide you toward an understanding of what some of these suggestions entail. The value in the discussion plan is the ability to review the details of some decisions ahead of time. Understanding the options in your birth space can help you make meaningful choices surrounding your labor and may help you decrease some of the anxiety related to childbirth.

BIRTH PLAN

Part two is the actual birth plan, which can be thought of as the final draft of your birth plan no matter where your chosen birth space is. The decisions in your birth plan should now be aligned with what your provider understands as feasible and safe for your particular labor. After some days, weeks, or months of scribbling out areas of your discussion plan, clarifying options, having introspective time, and becoming informed about the various options available at your birth place, you now have the plan you will present. Preferably during the last few weeks of pregnancy, you should put copies of the final draft of your birth plan in a central and visible location, such as on the refrigerator, as a sign you have prepared and are ready to bring your baby into the world on your terms.

Your succinct birth plan is comprehensive enough to serve as a map, or a reference guide as to which chosen birth space will work best over another. Choosing a birthplace that reflects your understanding of the laboring process, your unique comfort level, and your vision for labor is important. While one person may prefer a comfortable, home-like environment, another may prefer the routine and options available at a hospital. As the anxiety and excitement of a new baby draws near, it can be easy to forget the details of how and why a certain space was chosen to labor. Your birth plan acts as a supplement to your voice when you are busy doing important physical and mental labor. I suggest that your birth plan be used as a visual cue, and as a reminder to anyone occupying your birth space, of the work, discussion, thought, self-discovery, self-advocacy, and purpose you have put into the last portion of your pregnancy.

Birth Plan Basics

While every birth plan is going to be different because of varying goals and experiences, the basic components of a successful birth plan are the same. Your job, as you go through each section, is to understand what different birth spaces can accommodate. This understanding will lead you to the decisions that feel right for you.

ON ARRIVAL

This section of your birth plan will serve to introduce you to people unfamiliar with you or who are just meeting you for the first time. Your legal name (and what you prefer to be called), date of birth, pronouns, due date, provider, and your baby's pediatrician should be in a clearly visible space. Also include the names and contact numbers of all the members of your birth team who plan to be with you in your birth space. Note that your support team should be contacted upon your arrival to the birth space if you are not in the position to notify them on your own.

ATMOSPHERE

This section of the birth plan goes into detail about the environment and mood you would like to create in your labor and birth space. You will decide on lighting, music, focal points, aromatherapies, and any other tools to create an inviting and comfortable ambiance for you to labor in.

LABOR PREFERENCES

This section of the birth plan is the most detailed part of the plan and covers everything from induction, positioning, pain management specific to labor, and monitoring.

PAIN MANAGEMENT

Additional options for pain management and whether you will be offered interventions are included in this section of the birth plan. You will name the person you would like to be in charge of offering pain-relieving strategies, or you can designate yourself as the person in charge of asking for your preferred specific pain-management option. As you go through each option, remember that the birth plan allows for plenty of lenience, should you choose to make these decisions in real time.

SPECIAL TECHNIQUES, MONITORING THE BABY, AND CERVICAL EXAMS

If you have taken a childbirth education series that uses signature techniques, such as the Bradley method, HypnoBirthing, or Lamaze, that information should be indicated in this section of the birth plan. If you are not planning on using medication management as a coping strategy, be sure to indicate this preference in this section. If monitoring of your baby and contractions by continuous external fetal monitoring is not indicated, you should put this preference here. If you have preferences for if, when, and how you receive cervical exams, record these choices here as well.

BIRTH PREFERENCES

The birth preference section of the birth plan speaks to the start of the second stage of labor. You will indicate your plans for when it comes time to push in the second stage, including the positions you would like to try to push in and whether you would like a mirror to see external progression. Your decisions about the immediate period following the birth of the baby are also included in this section. This portion of the birth plan in real time goes by quickly and covers many small options.

EPISIOTOMY, CAESAREAN, AND ASSISTED VAGINAL BIRTHS

This birth plan section covers when and how your provider decides you would benefit from interventions to assist you in achieving a vaginal birth, such as an episiotomy or use of an assistive instrument such as vacuum or forceps. This section also handles such details of how a cesarean section would be accomplished if this procedure is determined necessary, including who you would like to accompany you during the procedure as well as what environment you would like during the procedure. This section also includes your wishes for the immediate care of your newborn in the operating room.

THIRD STAGE LABOR

Third stage and immediate newborn preferences, such as deciding on immediate skin-to-skin contact, are included in this section of the birth plan. The location of your birth should not change how you would like to handle your placenta. This section also details what is to be done for placental remains, and includes such options as allowing blood to cease pulsing prior to the umbilical cord being clamped and cut, or what to do with cord blood or placental tissue.

NEWBORN PREFERENCES

Choices regarding the care of your newborn will be outlined in this section. You will indicate whether you are planning a circumcision procedure to remove the foreskin of the penis during your hospital stay, or if you are planning medication or vaccine administration, or both. This section is also where you will indicate the timeline you would like these practices to be done.

HOSPITAL OR BIRTH CENTER STAY

This section of the birth plan covers your immediate and longer-term plans for your postpartum recovery, such as who plans on staying with you during your recovery. If you are not planning to labor and birth at home, you will indicate how long you would like to recover in the hospital or birth center, including plans for early discharge or if you'd like rooming-in. This space will outline your feeding plans. It is also where you will indicate if you would like to use services such as lactation support or help with newborn care basics such as bathing and diapering.

You will also note your religious or cultural practices here. Events such as circumcision or special traditions that require an additional person, or accommodations, should be mentioned

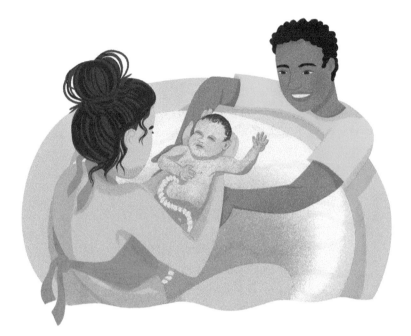

here. After you discuss your preferences with your pregnancy caregiver, have them sign the birth plan indicating you've discussed the plan with them so your wishes will be honored.

How to Imagine Your Perfect Childbirth Experience

Envision your perfect childbirth experience. This mental exercise is designed to help you uncover potential physical and emotional blockages that can impede your labor journey and assist you in drafting your birth plan. It will help you identify how to obtain the outcomes you envision. Begin this exercise starting at the end, when you are holding your baby. You have anticipated this moment for a long time and it has finally arrived. Are you smiling? Feel the weight of your baby in your arms and listen to their soft breathing. What do you feel? Looking to your side, who is with you? Is the space familiar? Do you have any items with you that bring you a sense of familiarity and comfort? How is the lighting? What do you hear? How is your body positioned? Are you sitting up in a bed? Are you dressed or naked? Discover what this moment looks like for you.

How did you get to here? Continue to navigate back to the moment your baby was born. What would feel right? Are you standing, squatting, laying on your back, or on your side? Are you in water, or have you settled into a space on the floor when your baby decidedly makes their appearance? Now go back even further. How did you labor? Was your team supportive and respectful? Dig deeper. Go back further into transition; you know this is the most difficult part. Is this intense portion what you expected? Does anything surprise or scare you? Continue navigating backward through labor, taking your time to uncover the details of where labor began, and how you alerted your birth team you were having contractions. Modify the visualization until you are able to draft your unique birth plan.

Ten Tips for Creating a Birth Plan

I offer you 10 tips on how to organize information, have difficult conversations, and accept difficult setbacks. As you develop your discussion plan, refer to this list while trying to remain on target for achieving your goals.

Jump around

Start filling in areas of the birth plan that come easily to you. These responses will help guide other decisions on the birth plan. For example, if you know you would like epidural anesthesia in labor, that will, by default, make other decisions obsolete, such as the use of IV pain medications or choosing whether you would even like an IV.

Find your alternatives

On occasion, you may have your mind set on a particular aspect of your labor only to find out that option is not feasible in your birth space. Ask your provider about alternatives. A client of mine was set on using the tub while she was in labor. She developed a condition that took away that option in the hospital space. Understanding what a wonderful tool hydrotherapy is for pain control, she agreed to use the shower as an alternative. She was disappointed that her original plan was not going to be an option, but discussion opened the gate for alternatives.

Know your policies

Some of your preferences may not be available or might be outside standard practice. Policies are not law, but be prepared to know what is and isn't standard in your chosen birth space. More important, know what you need to do when what you would like is not standard. A family I cared for wanted a lotus birth. The policy of the institution, which they provided to my client, stated that certain criteria would need to be met to allow this deviation from their standard newborn postpartum care. My client kept their policy as a reference alongside her birth plan, so there would be no difficulty in achieving the newborn care they desired.

Bring your discussion plan with you

Being prepared to go through your birth plan as a checklist throughout your pregnancy will help you and your provider identify ways to help you achieve your goals and uncover additional questions. One client of mine, week after week, brought in a rag-gedy, stained, written on, crossed out, and highlighted notebook that served as her discussion plan. Now, while I can't condone the appearance of this notebook, I can condone that she stayed on track week after week as questions came up, and plans were made as she prepared for her upcoming birth. In labor, she joked about how impressed I must be by her clear, unwrinkled, crisp birth plan on display in her labor room.

Make many copies

Once you have a finalized birth plan, make copies and put them in both conspicuous and unexpected places. Being able to access your birth plan electronically is also a good idea. Take a picture or send your support person an email. In fact, you may want to con-sider who of your labor support persons will be responsible for making sure the document is with you if your chosen birth space is not your home.

Make it your own

Cross it out. Feel free to modify any of the options. Make it personal and in alignment with what you want. Many of your decisions are based on generic standard available options. That doesn't mean that what you want is any less valid.

Select all or select none

If you don't particularly want an intervention, cross it out for emphasis. Likewise, if you feel like you are open for all of the available options, mark them all.

Rank your preferences

If you get to a portion of your birth plan where you have some options that are important, but you would prefer one option over another, rank these decisions in order of importance.

Keep it close

Be careful about who has access to your birth plan document. Consider only sharing your birth plan with members of your supportive birth team. The opinions of those not directly involved in your care and who will not be doing the physical work of labor are unneeded and unnecessary. Your birth plan is about your body, your choices, and your level of comfort. Your birth plan is not a document soliciting advice from others not involved in this process.

Post it in a conspicuous place

Post your birth plan. Doing so is a little different than just having several copies available. A birth plan in your bag or in a medical chart is not an effective way for those in your space to be mindful of the fact that you are an active participant in your and your baby's care. Your support person can help you find a location in your birth space that places the birth plan in an obnoxiously visible location for those present to reference as needed.

Who Should Review the Birth Plan?

Review your birth plan with the members of your support team, including your partner, doula, and anyone else you are planning to have in your birth space. When you have finalized the birth plan, it is helpful to have your provider sign it so anyone else coming in contact with you, or your written preferences, can understand you have the support of your provider.

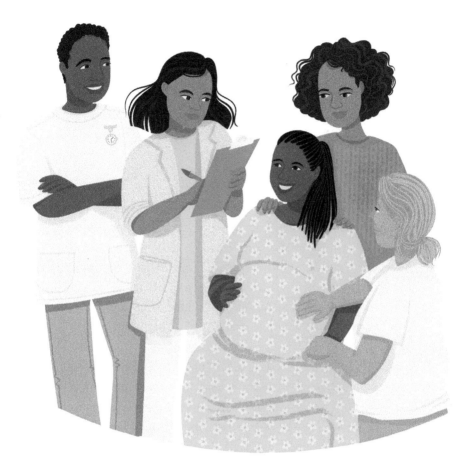

Also, consider how your support persons may operate in the birth space. It can be quite difficult to watch someone you love or care for be in pain or discomfort. Others may be uncomfortable with blood, nudity, or authority. It's important for your support to serve as a vocal advocate, if needed. Consider if this person can put aside their own discomfort to show up for you in a way that you need them to in your birth space. There is always a possibility that you choose someone unable to put aside their own discomforts and physical needs. When this occurs, their presence in your birth space could unintentionally divert attention away from your needs. Share your birth plan well ahead of time with the people you think you would like to have with you in labor.

BIRTH PLANS ARE NOT CONTRACTS

Regardless of the amount of time and attention you spend on your birth plan, it is in no way a legally binding document. Some providers will decline to honor birth plans. If this policy is identified during your prenatal care, it can be helpful that you reiterate your understanding of what a birth plan means to you: It is a written tool to help guide you toward decisions that are made about you, your labor, and your baby.

When framing a discussion about a birth plan with a provider who is not open to the idea, try to come to a common understanding that you both desire the safest birth outcomes. It is far easier to find common ground than to find a new provider. At any time during the pregnancy, if the pregnant person is unable to come to a consensus on how they would like to be cared for, or they do not feel supported, it is certainly reasonable to seek a new pregnancy care provider. Red flags include disregard for cultural practices, indifference about your queries or concerns, and any form of disrespect or abusive behavior. Any behavior you deem as a red flag is reason for finding a new provider.

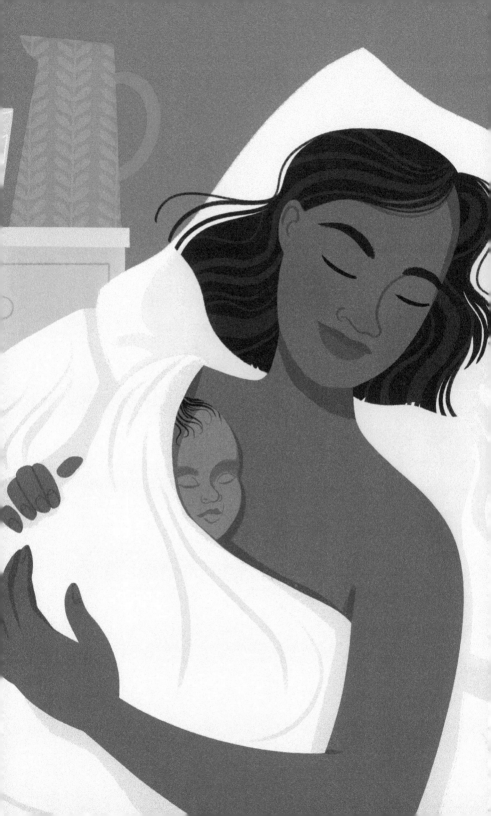

PART TWO

Building Your Birth Plan

Now that you've learned about birth preferences and options, it's time to build your birth plan. This section will help you prioritize your choices and organize your plan. You will learn more about the specifics of hospital and birth center options and how they affect your birth preferences. By the end of this section, you will have the tools to help you complete the birth plan template at the end of the book (see page 132). Putting your choices in writing will help you feel more comfortable and confident in sharing your birth plan with your support team.

Chapter 4

Before Childbirth

A large portion of your pregnancy may very well be the preparations you make for childbirth. Decisions about where you choose to birth and how you would like to receive your education often go hand in hand. Some people prefer a self-study approach, whereas others would like to be fully guided in a childbirth education series as they lean more on formalized classes with instructors. Your personal preferences will help you make the best decisions to suit your needs during this time.

BIRTH STORY: A MIDWIFE'S PERSPECTIVE

Stating your labor plans is always a good starting point to help you prepare for and reach your goals. Fiona was certain of her desire to labor for as long as she could without the use of interventions, namely epidural anesthesia. As she began to think about her goal, the bigger question became: How will I prepare for laboring as long as I can without the use of an epidural? Fiona enrolled in a class that emphasized techniques of self-hypnosis to facilitate relaxation and the elimination of physical and mental fear to allow her to progress through labor without intervention. As she began to learn more, she was faced with conflicting messages. She needed one unifying message: that she could labor and birth without interventions. Full stop. This message evolved through the process of creating a birth vision and plan.

Another client, Geraldine, had goals outside accepted norms for a first-time laborer. She was sure beyond all doubt that she would like to have a primary elective cesarean section. She had come to this decision for personal reasons that existed long before conception. Mostly, she was not interested in any interference in her plan, including hearing or talking about reasons an elective cesarean section is generally not ideal. What she was looking for was someone to support her decision. As the prenatal course continued, Geraldine's birth date was decided on with a scheduled cesarean section. The institutional rules for a surgical birth meant Geraldine could only have one support person with her in the operating room. Although Geraldine had wanted both her parents and partner with her, the hierarchy of decisions found its importance in the birthing method she wanted rather than in needing all members of her desired support team present.

Both women placed themselves in a good position for realizing their birth plans by considering their hierarchy of needs. Fiona needed tools to help her accomplish her plan of a non-medicated birth, then she needed a team that understood she was using a particular strategy that would require as little external interference as possible as she instituted her learned techniques during her labor and birth process. Understanding the roles and types of support Geraldine and Fiona were each going to have was critical in both of these women's births. Whatever you envision for your birth, the most satisfactory birth experiences are those in which people are informed about their choices and make plans that are in alignment with what they want.

Birth Centers Versus Hospitals Versus Home Births

Choosing a location is perhaps the most significant decision you can make in developing your birth plan. The options available for you for a home birth or at a birth center or hospital birth will help guide your labor and birth decisions. Remember Geraldine, who wanted a surgical birth? She understood that her goal would require her to give birth in a hospital. The same conclusions can be made for those who would like epidural anesthesia—an out-of-hospital experience is not a goal in this situation. Likewise, some choose their birth place based on the ability to have a certain number of support team members present. Your hierarchy of needs is a way to understand the options available to you in your chosen birth space. The easiest deciding factor can simply be the desire for an intervention not available in a particular space.

Hospitals

The majority of people choose to labor and birth in hospitals. Your hospital stay durations will vary, but standard time is one to two days following an uncomplicated vaginal delivery, and two to three days following an uncomplicated cesarean section. The industrialization of birth during the turn of the 21st century was driven largely by a promise of a pain-free birthing experience, and this can be seen today with rates of epidurals upward of 90 percent in hospitals. There is also a higher volume of labor and birth. To manage this increase, interventions that would not normally occur in non-hospital birth spaces are seen as the default. For example, common interventions, such as continuous external fetal monitoring or the administering of IV fluids, are common but may not always be needed. People trust hospital environments because of the security of being surrounded by a wide range of providers and resources. It's important to know what various interventions accomplish and which are necessary for one's own birth preferences.

Understanding the policies of your hospital birth space, and knowing who will be providing your care there, will allow you to develop a birth plan in line with what the facility is able to offer, and to develop a plan more closely in line with your goals for labor and birth. Presenting to your birth space as an informed consumer is the best thing you can do to ensure that the vision you have for your birth is not superseded by your chosen birth environment. A birth plan that reflects your realistic options shows that you are an educated healthcare consumer. Your birth plan provides you an opportunity to demonstrate you are not rejecting hospital standardized care; rather, you are an active participant in individualized care for you and your baby. Choosing a hospital birth doesn't mean just following the provided path; it's important to be an informed participant to meet the goals of your birth. The next section will give you more guidance.

Hospital tours give you the option to assess a facility for your own needs. Use these questions as a starting place and feel free to make a list of a few questions personal to your birth preferences. Because a variety of people are employed to guide hospital tours, be ready to ask what their role is.

✛ **Where do I go when I am in labor?**
You don't realize how many doors hospitals have until you are in active labor and just trying to get in the building. Some hospitals have different entrances for those in labor versus those with medical emergencies.

✛ **Where do I park?**
Ask all the parking questions you can think of, including visitor parking, towing, and alternative options. Consider the cost of parking to get the instructions you need to avoid parking costs.

✛ **Is there any time during the check-in process when I will be asked to separate from my labor support people?**
The answer to this question may guide some of your preferences as you develop a birth plan.

✛ **Who can I expect to see when I am getting assessed for labor in the hospital?**
You may see a nurse or providers such as a doctor or midwife. Ask if providers are on site 24-7 or if you can request a particular provider.

+ **Are some members of the hospital team there in a learning capacity, such as medical students, midwifery students, or resident physicians?**
This answer will allow you to understand who the standard members of the care teams are in the hospital. If you don't mind learners, but would prefer they only observe your birth space, you can ask how that is accomplished.

+ **Can I wear my own clothes?**
This answer will advise you of standard hospital protocol, and help you consider other options outside the standard in your birth plan.

+ **Does the hospital provide any labor support tools?**
Some options, like nitrous oxide, are available only in hospitals or birth centers, but a facility may have other tools such as exercise balls, rebozos, peanut balls, massage instruments, TENS units, and hydrotherapy-like pools, showers, and tubs. For options that you want but are not available, ask if you can bring in your own tools from home.

+ **Are there any policies that would restrict the use of hydrotherapy while in labor?**
Some hospital policies allow for the use of hydrotherapy in labor but restrict it during birth.

+ **Is there a designated anesthesia team on site to perform epidurals?**
In some hospitals, anesthesiologists are shared with other areas of the hospital, while others have anesthesiologists designated for labor and delivery units.

✤ What are your epidural policies?
Understand the administration of this intervention and if
there is a time that's considered "too late" for an epidural.

✤ Can I bring food from home to eat?
Ask about the storage of food and beverages, too.

✤ How many births take place each month?
What's the cesarean birth rate? The national average for
surgical birth is around 30 percent; some facilities have
higher or lower than average rates. Although it is impossible
to draw any conclusions from a hospital's birth rate, knowing
your chosen hospital's cesarean birth rates in comparison
to the national average may be something to consider when
choosing a particular facility.

✤ What are the visitor policies?
This response will help you decide who will be present in the
delivery room and who can stay with you. You will also learn
designated times for visitation after delivery.

✤ What is the rooming-in policy?
Rooming-in information tells you where infants are in
proximity to their parents during the in-hospital postpartum
stay. This answer will help you understand if the standard
hospital policies are in alignment with how you would like
to room.

✤ Are there postpartum amenities?
These amenities include lactation support as well as infant
care classes during your stay.

Some essentials will be provided to you during your hospital stay. You do not need to worry about hydration or what to wear during labor. However, you may want to bring items that will assist you through labor if the hospital does not have them available. You won't need to worry about standard postpartum supplies like disposable underwear, peri-bottle, and pads, but consider what happens after the baby comes. In most cases, you will recover overnight for a few days, so bring comfortable clothes that will facilitate chest-feeding and skin-to-skin contact, and don't forget yourself. If you have specialized hygiene or skin care items, bring them from home. Below are some suggestions for additional items to put in your hospital birth kit.

- **Preferred Beverages (and method to maintain their temperature, if needed)**
  - Check with your hospital to see if there are restrictions on the types of beverages you may consume while admitted in labor
  - Electrolyte popsicles
  - Fresh fruit including lemon/lime slices
  - Honey sticks

- **Labor Tools (if your hospital does not provide them)**
  - Aromatherapy
  - Device to play music or sounds
  - Exercise balls
  - Gum or hard candy (ask about hospital restrictions)
  - Handheld fan
  - Lip balm
  - Massage oil

- [ ] Massagers (electric or manual)
- [ ] TENS unit
- [ ] Warming and cooling packs

Daily Personal Hygiene

- [ ] Hair dryer
- [ ] Herbal perineal treatments
- [ ] Large overnight pads
- [ ] Quality soap, shampoo, conditioner, toothpaste, etc.
- [ ] Underwear (cotton) to support hospital underwear with possibly heavy perineal packs

Comfort Items

- [ ] Blanket
- [ ] Chargers
- [ ] Easy-on-and-off pajamas
- [ ] Pillows for chest-feeding and comfort
- [ ] Robe
- [ ] Slippers with grip
- [ ] Socks

Birth Centers

Birth centers in the United States represent the standard of care for low-risk labor and birth, although only 0.3 percent of U.S. births occur in birth centers. A birth center, although equipped to handle most birth emergencies on site, is unable to perform surgical births. The goal of a birth center is to mimic a home-like environment and contain many of the amenities that would make birth comfortable. Many people like that birth centers do not share the same restrictions, such as who can accompany you during labor, as industrialized birth settings. Hydrotherapy, in the form of showers and ergonomic tubs or pools, allow immersion during labor and are accommodating enough for birth. Birth centers utilize local anesthetics but not epidurals, and some may provide IV pain medication or inhaled analgesics, such as nitrous oxide, for pain control.

The birth center will not have freely exposed medical equipment or continuous external fetal monitors. The standard of care for fetal monitoring is done intermittently throughout the different phases of labor using a hand-held doppler or fetoscope. Expect birth assistants, nurses, midwifery students, and  primarily midwives for your birth team. Midwives are experts in low-intervention, normal, healthy labor and birth. Individuals with conditions that put their pregnancy at risk typically cannot labor and birth at birth centers. It is for this and many reasons that birth centers generally have cesarean birth rates ranging from 3 to 6 percent. The most common non-emergency reason for transferring from a birth center to a hospital is to seek pain control.

The postpartum recovery at a birth center differs from hospital births, and one can expect to stay anywhere from 6 to 24 hours following birth. You would treat your stay like an Airbnb. Typical amenities will be present, but you will want to bring in items that would make your stay more comfortable, including your preferred foods and beverages. Many centers will have basic postpartum hygiene care items available, but prepare to purchase any specialty postpartum recovery care items, such as perineal packs, pads, and peri-bottles to take with you as you continue your recovery at home. Becoming more informed about your birth place options will help you be confident in your choices when considering how much comfort you want during labor.

Touring a birth center lets you experience the environment and see how it fits with your birth preferences. Aside from essential questions, such as whether they accept your health insurance, it's important to talk to your guide and assess their role in that space. The following questions, in addition to ones that you come up with on your own, should serve as a foundation:

+ **Is this birth center part of a larger hospital system?**
Birth centers can be part of a larger hospital system—even located inside hospitals—or freestanding. Knowing whether the birth center is hospital-based may influence some of your options as you develop your birth plan.

+ **Is the birth center accredited by any governing body?**
Accreditation comes from organizations such as the Commission for the Accreditation of Birth Centers (CABC), which has very specific requirements for accreditation. Some birth centers are not accredited by CABC but *are* licensed by the state. If birth center accreditation is important to you and the site is not accredited, you may want to ask why to determine whether this information will factor into your choice.

+ **Do you carry any liability insurance?**
   In many states, providers are required to carry insurance as a protection for themselves and their clients.

+ **Do you take my health insurance?**
   In many states, birth center births are not a covered service. If the financial component of having a birth center birth is a deciding factor, ask about payment plans, or if there is an alternative means for covering services.

+ **What if I'm in labor and a space is not available?**
   Ask how many births occur per month and how many birth suites are in the facility. The answer will indicate the likelihood you would need a backup option.

+ **Are there members of the birth center team who are in the facility in a learning capacity, such as nursing or midwifery students?**
   This answer will allow you to understand who the standard members of the care teams are and who you may expect to see at your birth.

+ **What type of labor support tools are available?**
   Many birth centers have the option of using nitrous oxide during labor. They may also supply exercise balls, rebozos, peanut balls, massage instruments, TENS units, and hydrotherapy-like pools, showers, and tubs. For options that you want but are not available, ask if you can bring in your own tools from home.

+ What are some reasons I would transfer to the hospital?
Planning an out-of-hospital birth or a planned home birth
does not mean you stay out of the hospital no matter what.
For out-of-hospital births, understand which instances will
result in a decision to transfer to the hospital.

**+ What are the birth center–to–hospital transfer
arrangements?**
If a hospital transfer is needed, know how you will get there
and whether your midwife will still be involved in your care
in any capacity.

+ What is the postpartum timeline?
This answer will give you an idea of when you would be
discharged following birth so you can plan what to pack.

**+ How do you obtain your baby's birth certificate, and how
do you go about state-mandated newborn screening?**
After birth, some state-mandated newborn screenings will
be offered for your newborn. These screenings are obtained
24 to 48 hours after birth, so this timeline will determine
when the midwife comes to your home for the postpartum
visit and what, if anything, you need to do to obtain your
birth certificate.

BIRTH CENTER BIRTH KIT

Remember that a birth center will mimic a home and will include
rudimentary hygiene items and toiletries in the same way that
hospital settings will. Birth centers will also have a kitchen for
your food items. Bring the items that comfort you from your own

space. Like hospitals, birth centers have basic items available for labor tools, but you will likely want to prepare for the personalization of your space. In addition to all the ways you make your home comfortable for yourself on a regular day, focus on the tools of labor and the immediate postpartum period.

- Preferred Beverages and Foods: Focus on items easily transported to and from the birth center with minimal hassle and preparation.
  - ☐ Electrolyte popsicles
  - ☐ Fresh fruit including lemon/lime slices
  - ☐ Honey sticks

- Labor Tools (see what is available at the birth center)
  - ☐ Aromatherapy
  - ☐ Device to play music or sounds
  - ☐ Exercise balls
  - ☐ Gum or hard candy
  - ☐ Handheld fan
  - ☐ Lip balm
  - ☐ Massage oil
  - ☐ Massagers (electric or manual)
  - ☐ TENS unit
  - ☐ Warming and cooling packs

- Daily Personal Hygiene (immediate postpartum period)
  - ☐ Large overnight pads
  - ☐ Herbal perineal treatments
  - ☐ Quality soap, shampoo, conditioner, toothpaste, etc.
  - ☐ Underwear to support disposable underwear with possibly heavy perineal packs

Comfort Items

- ☐ Chargers
- ☐ Easy-on-and-off pajamas
- ☐ Pillows for chest-feeding and comfort
- ☐ Robe
- ☐ Slippers with grip
- ☐ Socks

Home Birth

A planned home birth with a qualified provider such as a midwife or physician is a safe and reasonable option for low-risk individuals. The largest benefit of giving birth at home is being able to be in your own space, as a master of your comfort and domain. Midwives who provide home birth services follow the same standard of care for low-risk people in labor as do the providers at a birth center or hospital by using intermittent auscultation (listening for the patterns in the fetal heart rate in relationship to contractions) with the use of a doppler or fetoscope as the method of fetal assessment in labor. Being the expert in your space, you are only limited in labor by what you feel comfortable doing in your own home. People choosing home births generally have ideas about which part of the home they plan to use in labor as well as who they would like to accompany them in their space. Eating and drinking is encouraged throughout labor, if desired, and you can expect the rules of your home to dictate the rules of your birth space.

Planning a labor and birth at home means you will not have the options for pain control that are available in a birth center or hospital. If you think an epidural, IV pain medication, or inhaled analgesics are part of your birth plan, then a home birth is not a feasible option. Like birth center births, home births should be reserved for low-risk individuals. Your home birth provider will carry emergency equipment and medication to your home and will determine through strict criteria who is best suited for low-intervention labor and birth. Ultimately, your home is not the hospital and does not have the level of intervention to support an emergency that would require surgery or assisted vaginal deliveries. Understanding your absence of risk factors is a critical first step in determining whether a home birth is a good option for you.

QUESTIONS WHEN CONSIDERING HOME BIRTH

Most of the questions to ask before considering home birth will start with you and how comfortable you are in your home. Also, look for a reliable, qualified provider who takes your health insurance (or find out what the costs will be) who will care for you. The questions that follow, along with any others, should lead the discussion when speaking to a potential provider about a home birth.

+ **Are you licensed to practice home births in the state?**
  This may or may not be a deal breaker, depending on the state where you live. For example, some states do not have any legislation regarding midwifery, yet midwifery is alive and well. Other states have regulations restricting certain types of midwives from practicing in hospitals, while others restrict the practice of other types of midwifery outside hospitals. The absence or presence of a license may be a determining factor in whether you proceed with a home birth at all.

+ **Do you carry any liability insurance?**
  Many states require home birth midwives to carry liability insurance. Liability insurance protects midwives and others in the event the person in their care is injured or there are

damages. Reasons vary as to why a midwife may not have liability insurance. If having this insurance is important to you, ask about it.

✤ **Can you evaluate the space I would like to birth in?**
Providers may have feedback about the feasibility of using a particular space, especially a bathtub.

✤ **Will the midwife bring any additional members for support?**
Many home birth midwives serve multiple roles as care providers, educators, and preceptors to student midwives. Having students be part of the birth team is not uncommon. If a student may be present, you may want to know ahead of time.

✤ **What are the birth center–to–hospital transfer arrangements?**
If a hospital transfer is needed, know how you will get there and whether your midwife will still be involved in your care in any capacity.

✤ **Will I need to obtain any medication for the birth on my own?**
Depending on the laws in your state, your provider may bring their own medications or prescriptions, or both, or you may need to have prescription medications picked up at a local pharmacy as part of your home birth kit.

✤ **What is the postpartum timeline with regard to the midwife's stay?**
Following a home birth, midwives generally stay for a few hours after the birth. Generally speaking, you can expect a

postpartum visit within 24 to 48 hours as well. Providers' postpartum visit schedule will vary.

✛ **How many other labors do you oversee in a month and what are the arrangements for stand-ins?**
If you and another patient are in labor simultaneously, the stand-in provider would then become a member of your birth team. If it is important to you to meet this person "just in case," ask about an opportunity to get to know the stand-in provider ahead of time.

✛ **How will newborn screening be accomplished?**
Within the 24-to-48-hour mark, the baby will be offered state-mandated testing for the most common genetic and metabolic disorders. Some midwives do this testing, while other home birth midwives will defer this testing to the pediatrician. The same goes for obtaining the birth certificate. Some midwives will handle all the paperwork, while others will leave obtaining the birth certificate up to you.

HOME BIRTH KIT

Your provider will bring instruments for monitoring you and your baby, such as a fetoscope or doppler, a blood pressure cuff, thermometer, and pulse oximeter. The provider will also supply various medical materials, such as scissors, cord clamps, measuring tapes, and a portable scale, in addition to sterile supplies like syringes for medication administration, gloves, antiseptic solutions, and assorted absorptive materials. Emergency equipment, such as oxygen and neonatal resuscitation supplies, will also be brought into the home.

Your home birth provider will advise you of the items they would like you to have available at your home for your labor and birth. If anything needs to be purchased, your midwife may direct you to preferred vendors to purchase these specialty items designed specifically for those planning a home birth. Kits will vary, but most will include items for the immediate postpartum period, such as peri-bottles, disposable underwear, assorted under pads, a disposable bulb syringe, and gauze. Additional items, already in your home, that should bring you comfort and familiarity include:

▨ Preferred Beverages and Food: Focus on stocking your refrigerator with several beverage options and packing your freezer with low-prep foods.

▨ Labor and Birth Tools (check to see what your midwife or doula supplies)

☐ Large glass or plastic bowl for placenta
☐ Handheld or electric fan
☐ Flashlight, extra batteries
☐ Large black garbage bags
☐ Gallon-size, resealable plastic bags
☐ Extra bed sheets
☐ Large shower curtain to place under your sheets to protect your mattress
☐ Large towels (several and may get stained)
☐ Wash cloths (several and may get stained)
☐ If you are purchasing a portable tub, remember the under-tarp, food-grade hose that can reach the tub, and the pump to remove water.

■ Personal Hygiene and Comfort Items (postpartum period)

☐ Preferred footwear
☐ Large overnight sanitary pads
☐ Herbal perineal treatments
☐ Easy-on-and-off pajamas
☐ Pillows for chest-feeding and comfort
☐ Robe
☐ Underwear (cotton) that can support wearing heavy perineal packs

Your Childbirth Team

For those planning for a vaginal birth, begin assembling a team to assist you as soon as you can. This section will help you highlight people who may have various roles in your pregnancy, labor, and birth. Some of the decisions you make about who to include as members of your team will impact your ability to carry out the type of labor and birth plan you desire. For example, someone who prefers an OB/GYN as a pregnancy care provider may have difficulty using a birth center or delivering at home because of where obstetricians practice. Depending on the environment you choose, you may be limited in how many people you can have as part of your support team. The people in your labor and birth space can provide support and validation, and they can help facilitate your labor. Conversely, the presence of individuals who do not understand your vision can cause obstructions. This section will explain some of the central individuals commonly present during pregnancy, labor, and birth. Understanding the different roles of doulas, midwives, obstetricians, and your partner is key to understanding how each of these people support you through pregnancy and throughout labor and birth.

DOULAS

DOULAS

The number of things a doula can do for you when you are in labor could fill an entire book. This individual is hired by you as a non-medical member of your team to provide one-on-one labor support, but they are not a replacement for your partner or chosen support person. Doulas are primarily independent contractors, so how they operate their businesses and what services they offer will vary from person to person. Some doulas are trained using an apprentice model, while others obtain certifications through a doula certifying body and completion of in-person training that includes attendance at a specified number of births. A doula will do more than just serve as your cheerleader during labor. They also help implement the tools you learned in prenatal education. Exceptional doulas will advocate for your needs and preferences during labor and birth, as occasions necessitate. Some doulas have expanded their scope to include postpartum services such as breast- or chest-feeding support and newborn care.

How you will work with a doula will differ based on where you are planning to labor. Most doulas will meet you during your pregnancy and may work with you on many components of your birth plan to determine how they will be able to assist you in meeting your birth preferences. If you plan to give birth in a birth center or hospital, the ideal time to transition to your birth space is during active labor. You should expect a doula to be available to support you prior to going to your birth space and to remain with you for some time after you have your baby. If you are planning a hospital birth, check whether they require that persons serving as a doula need to be certified by a particular agency. Not all

doulas assist labors in hospitals, and not all doulas assist people at out-of-hospital births, so it is important to vet your doula to see if they will be able to assist you in meeting your labor and birth goals in your chosen birth space.

✛ **Are there any materials for me to review that outline the types of services you provide?**
Reviewing your prospective doula's materials will give you an opportunity to see if their specialties, experience, and offerings are in alignment with what you would like.

✛ **How much are your services?**
Find out the costs of the doula's services upfront so you can make necessary arrangements.

✛ **Do you hold any certifications and, if so, from which organizations?**
If they do not hold any certifications, ask about their apprenticeship training. If certification for some organizing body is important to you, ask about these affiliations.

✛ **How many times will I meet with you prior to going into labor?**
Each doula is different, including how they run their business. Part of what makes doula work beneficial for people in labor is the relationship they develop with their doula throughout their pregnancy.

✛ Will you accompany me to a third trimester prenatal appointment?
Doulas appreciate the opportunity to ask questions of and build working relationships with your labor support providers.

✛ How long have you been an independent doula?
Experience is important, but sometimes quality references reveal more about a doula than the number of births they have attended, though you will want to know both number of births and settings of those births. You want someone who will be a good fit for your birth plan.

✛ How long will you stay with me after delivery?
Some doulas specialize in postpartum aftercare; others do not. If they do provide postpartum care, ask about breast- or chest-feeding support. You may continue to have supportive needs in the postpartum period. Asking about the postpartum services may determine if you need to consider getting additional support.

✛ Is there a backup person to stand in if you're unable to attend my labor?
Doulas sometimes have multiple clients. Ask this question so you can be comfortable in the event the stand-in becomes your attendant. Ask to meet the stand-in if one is available. Also, meeting the stand-in before labor may provide more assurance if your doula is away.

In the United States, midwives currently attend 10 percent of all labors and births. The March of Dimes and World Health Organization, as well as numerous studies, have all reiterated that midwifery care leads to improved maternal outcomes, a decreased need for interventions, decreased cesarean section rates, and improved rates of sustained breastfeeding, and has many other benefits for the birthing individual and infant when compared to the obstetric medical model of care. Midwives have varying degrees of training, backgrounds, and scopes of practice. Accessibility to different types of midwives, including whether they can prescribe medications, will vary depending on the state. Midwives also differ from one to the other in terms of whether they are an insurance provider and where and how they received their training.

Some of the midwife designations include Certified Nurse Midwives (CNMs), Certified Professional Midwives (CPMs), Direct Entry Midwives (DEMs), and traditional midwives. Certified Nurse Midwives (CNMs) are registered nurses who complete master's-degree-level training at an accredited college or university and go on to complete a national certification exam. In all states, CNMs primarily deliver babies at hospitals; in many states, they can deliver babies in birth centers or in people's homes as well. CNMs can work independently, alongside, in collaboration with, or under the supervision of a board-certified obstetrician depending on the state. Certified Midwives (CMs) possess a college degree not in nursing and receive specialized training at an accredited school before passing the same board certification exam as CNMs. CMs can practice in hospitals, birth centers, or in homes depending on state regulations. Certified Professional Midwives (CPMs) are not required to hold a college degree. They complete a clinical apprenticeship training under a licensed midwife and must pass a clinical evaluation and national certification exam. CPMs are independent practitioners allowed to practice in most states who deliver care in birth centers and homes. Direct Entry Midwives (DEMs) are also known as *licensed midwives* or less commonly as *registered midwives*. DEMs complete an apprenticeship along with state-approved midwifery education. Many states recognize the legality of DEMs and allow them to deliver care in birth centers or homes. Traditional midwives are trained through an apprenticeship model, sometimes by taking up the pregnancy support practices specific to their cultures, without using an institution, and consequently hold no licenses or certifications from the state. They primarily deliver care in people's homes.

QUESTIONS WHEN INTERVIEWING A MIDWIFE

As you consider what kind of midwife to invite to your birth team, you will need to consider your preferences and eventual labor environment. Some of the questions you ask your potential midwifery provider may depend upon where they practice. Ask about receiving care outside of pregnancy for wellness and gynecological visits. Many midwives see non-pregnant people throughout their patient's lifespan. Use the following questions along with those pertinent to your plan to determine the right fit.

✢ **What are your credentials? Could you provide references?**
If you are planning to birth outside a hospital, you may want to determine the type of midwife you are considering, and check to see if they have credentials or licensing in the state. Ask if they have references you can contact. This question is more relevant to midwives who attend out-of-hospital births.

+ Do you perform breech deliveries?
Some midwife providers are skilled at delivering babies in
a multitude of presentations, whereas others are not. The
response to this question will shed light on what would occur
if your baby is not head down.

+ Are you certified in neonatal resuscitation (NPR)?
Five to 10 percent of infants will need some sort of help,
such as providing tactile stimulation like drying them
with a towel, to begin breathing and transition. Midwives
should be up to date on certification to show they have been
trained to perform resuscitation, if needed, as best practices
change often.

+ What services will my insurance cover?
Hospital midwifery services are typically covered by
insurance. If you are considering an out-of-hospital birth
with a midwife, ask about insurance and whether their
services are covered.

**+ How long have you been in practice and how many babies do
you deliver in a month?**
For larger volume practices, you may consider asking who else
could potentially attend your birth in the event the provider
is unavailable.

+ What's the cesarean section rate for you and your practice?
Ask if they know the cesarean section rate for their practice,
and for themselves personally.

+ **Will you be with me when I'm in in labor and have my baby?**
  Midwifery practices will vary on who will attend your labor.
  Determining factors depend on their birth space and volume
  of clients.

+ **Are there other types of providers who are part of the care
  team (OB/GYN residents, students)?**
  Ultimately, you should be aware of anyone who could
  potentially be in your birth space.

+ **What are your hospital transfer arrangements?**
  If you are considering an out-of-hospital birth, ask about
  hospital transfer arrangements and continuity of care if a
  transfer becomes necessary.

+ **Do you have hospital privileges?**
  For those planning an out-of-hospital birth, in the event
  a transfer becomes necessary, midwives with hospital
  privileges can continue to be part of the care team at
  the hospital.

+ **What's your philosophy as a midwife?**
  The answer to this question will help you better understand
  how your midwife's practices, training, experiences, and even
  individual nuances inform their personal philosophy.

+ **What are your thoughts on birth plans?**
  Open-ended questions will allow you to understand your
  provider's thoughts about using a concrete tool such as a birth
  plan to help you make informed and autonomous decisions.

+ **What are your thoughts on doulas?**
  Many midwives work with doulas on a regular basis. Your
  midwife may also have recommendations for doulas they have
  worked with.

+ **Do you have an expanded scope of practice that includes
  assisted vaginal deliveries?**
  If an assisted vaginal delivery becomes necessary, it is
  important to know if the midwife is able to perform
  this procedure.

OBSTETRICIANS

Obstetricians are medical specialists of pregnancy, childbirth,
and the postpartum period. They are the experts in managing,
treating, and evaluating complications and high-risk situations
that may occur throughout any of these periods. Obstetricians
are also gynecologists trained in surgical procedures related to
the gynecologic and reproductive systems, including cesarean
section births. Obstetricians in the United States are college
graduates who underwent additional medical school training,
completed a residency program, and passed medical board exams.
Many OB/GYNs have additional training for surgical specialties
and procedures. Most OB/GYNs deliver care in hospitals and
attend 90 percent of the births that occur there. A very small per-
centage of obstetricians attend births outside the hospital. Unlike
midwifery, obstetrical training is very similar regardless of where
you live. So, an important point to consider is the birth philosophy, temperament, and practices of each particular provider.

An obstetrician's approach will differ depending on where
they received their training, where they practice, and what their
personal philosophy is surrounding pregnancy, labor, and birth.

Labor and birth are intensive processes not only for the person having the baby, but also for those who support them in labor and attend their births. As the volume of laboring people increases, the less individual time your provider will be able to spend with you. In hospital settings with a higher volume of patients, this may mean that your obstetrician, with a higher patient load and other clinical and surgical responsibilities, would be less available to you as support in labor.

In collaborative practices, midwives and obstetricians care for many of the same patients, reserving OB/GYNs for high-risk patients, whose births may require more time and attention than those of individuals whose labor and births are low-risk and uncomplicated. This collaboration between midwives and OB/GYNs ensures they complement each other's work. The collaboration and division of patients in this manner reserves physicians for their other valuable skill sets, as needed.

QUESTIONS WHEN INTERVIEWING AN OBSTETRICIAN

Vetting your obstetrician will help you determine if they can be a member of your labor and birth team. Consider their personal philosophy surrounding labor and birth, birth plans, and intervention to see if you are a good match. Consider these questions in addition to other open-ended queries that may strike you as important.

✛ **Have you worked with clients who have used birth plans?** Birth plans are commonly recognized as a tool to communicate your labor and birth preferences. Your provider may have experience with how these tools work best and specific suggestions about how to use your birth plan in the birth space.

+ **Do you have experience working with doulas?**
Providers who have working relationships with doulas
can provide a recommendation and will understand the
important roles doulas play for the laboring person.

+ **Do you know the cesarean section rate for your practice, and
for yourself personally?**
Whereas facility and provider cesarean birth rates are not
predictive of your birth outcomes, having this information
may inform your choice of a provider.

+ **Will you be with me when I am in labor and have my baby?**
The volume of clients, structure of the practice, and how often
your provider is at the hospital will determine the likelihood
that your chosen obstetrician will be the person attending
your birth.

+ **Are there other types of providers part of the care team
(midwives, residents, or students)?**
You are always in charge of who is in your birth space, and
how involved you prefer those people to be. Knowing this
information will help you curate your birth space accordingly.

+ **What is your personal philosophy surrounding labor
and birth?**
The provider's responses will help determine if your
philosophies are a match.

+ **Have you worked with clients who use a birth plan?**
Ask an open-ended question about your choice to use a
birth plan.

+ Do you have an expanded scope of practice that includes breech deliveries?

Babies come out in a variety of positions. Not every obstetrician will delivery a baby in a position other than head first. Ask what their recommendation would be in the event your baby is breech near term.

+ Do you perform assisted vaginal deliveries?

When assistance is needed to accomplish a vaginal delivery, not all providers will use vacuum or forceps. They might have a preference for one or the other. This information is just good to know.

+ How do you handle the situation if I remain pregnant past my predicted due date?

The reponse to this question may help you identify providers who routinely offer elective inductions, or others who take a more conservative approach, after the estimated due date has passed.

YOUR PARTNER AS LABOR COACH

For those who are partnered, it is important to discuss how your partner envisions themselves as a participant in your labor and birth. Ideally, how you would like to see their role and how they would like to see their role are the same. If you are expecting them to be an active participant while they would prefer to be a bystander, if would be wise to address these expectations well in advance of labor. If you choose to have your partner included in your physical labor and birth space, at minimum it is helpful for them to understand what your goals are for their participation.

Partners as labor coaches should feel comfortable having a more physical, active, and primary role in your labor and birth process. For partners who want to play an active role, there are prenatal classes to help them be as supportive as possible. Specific courses of instruction, such as the Bradley method, focus on educating the partner to serve in the role of the primary labor support person, whereas other prenatal education programs, like the Lamaze technique, do not emphasize the partner as the sole labor coach and support person. When deciding on a labor coach, it's important to study and discuss the process and think through ways your coach can be effective. Your partner is in a unique position to be a huge asset for you during your labor because they know you better than the others on the team.

QUESTIONS TO ASK YOUR PARTNER

When you begin discussions with your partner about their own goals, the questions are quite different than those you would ask a prospective member of your birth team. Communication with your partner is vital to the successful implementation of your birth plan. Use these questions as a guideline or prompt to determine the questions you will ask your partner on your own. You know and understand your partner, but my hope is that these questions lead to conversations. Remember, the goal of these conversations is to understand your partner's thoughts and relay your own ideas to them.

+ **What are your thoughts about labor and birth? Does any part of it worry you?**
  Discuss your planned birth environment and your partner's feelings about the process.

✤ **How do you think you will feel seeing me uncomfortable?**
It's important to gauge and discuss your partner's possible reactions to the labor process.

✤ **Are you interested in taking prenatal education classes with me?**
Learning about pregnancy and labor will help you and your partner feel more confident during labor, but it's important to know if your partner wants to learn with you.

✤ **How do you visualize us and our space during labor and on the day of the birth?**
Ask your partner if they have thought about how they see themselves in that space on your labor and birth day.

✤ **How do you feel about the active or passive role you will be taking on?**
If your goals include your partner taking on a more active or physical role, ask them what their thoughts are about this. If your goals include your partner being more of a bystander, ask them what their thoughts are about this.

✤ **How do you feel about the other members of the birth team and their roles?**
If you are planning to enlist a doula as labor support, ask your partner what they know about doulas and how they feel about this choice.

Childbirth Education Classes

For many people, prenatal visits simply do not allow enough time for a reasonable education on preparing for labor and birth. Childbirth education classes can help you make smart decisions that will fit your preferences: deciding what type of birth you'd like to accomplish, who should assume what roles, and even what environment suits your needs best.

For those who would like to labor and birth without medication, childbirth education may help you discover methods and tools to make the experience manageable and tolerable. Labor is hard and uncomfortable. Your medication-free plan will flounder if you don't understand your options and have realistic expectations. In many cases, childbirth education is not covered by insurance. Classes vary widely in their philosophy, scope, and type of instructor, as do their costs and time commitment.

LAMAZE TECHNIQUE CLASSES

The Lamaze philosophy is founded on the belief that people have the instinctive ability to carry out the normal physiological processes of labor and birth. This technique supports people birthing wherever they deem appropriate for them and their families. Lamaze uses certified teachers, so you can expect a standard curriculum. This particular technique rose to popularity in the 1960s based on observations of Dr. Fernand Lamaze, who emphasized the methods people used to cope with labor as an alternative to using medicine for pain relief. Lamaze focuses on using tools to facilitate movement as well as relaxation for pain management through breathing techniques as opposed to pain elimination. Those using Lamaze techniques may decide to forgo pain medication in favor of their learned techniques, whereas others may plan to use medication or an epidural for pain control. Wanting to have an unmedicated labor is not a requirement of being able to benefit from Lamaze. These classes are typically held in person for a period of six to eight weeks, meeting once a week for around 12 total hours of instruction. Some classes can be taken over the course of a weekend. Many hospital-based education programs, although not officially certified by Lamaze, are structured around many of the Lamaze techniques for coping with pain.

THE BRADLEY METHOD CLASSES

This method focuses on a medication- and anesthesia-free birth. The Bradley method relies on one's partner as the primary support person in labor. The Bradley method was founded in the 1940s by an American obstetrician, Robert Bradley, and the instruction accentuates the role of diet and exercise as part of labor preparation throughout pregnancy. You can expect this course to last 12 weeks, combining a mix of in-person teaching with some variation of homework, taught by certified instructors. This philosophy works by implementing the methods learned about relaxation, releasing tension, releasing fear, and receiving the coaching instruction the partner provides throughout labor. Patients who plan to have a medication-free birth and a primary labor partner will benefit most from this method.

HYPNOBIRTHING CLASSES

HypnoBirthing, less commonly referred to as the Mongen method, was first recognized in the late 1980s when the technique was described in a book by the nurse Michelle Leclaire O'Neill.

HypnoBirthing is built on the premise that learning breathing techniques, visualization, and meditation as a method to increase endorphins and release the effects of stress hormones that increase our perceptions of pain will serve as a substitute for the use of medications as pain control. These classes are taught by individuals who have been certified by the organization HypnoBirthing International. Classes are taught in five 2½ hour courses and include in-person classes and a fair level of personal introspection and commitment to implement learned labor techniques. HypnoBirthing relies on having your other support persons know you are implementing HypnoBirthing techniques and considers how they can support you best. A deep meditative state can be interrupted by well-meaning individuals who do not understand the process of HypnoBirthing.

EVIDENCE BASED BIRTH CLASSES

Evidence Based Birth is an analytical approach to labor and birth with a goal to use research and evidence to support labor and birth goals. It was established in 2015 by Dr. Rebecca Decker after her own childbirth experience left her evaluating gaping holes in the care she received. Evidence Based Birth instructors have been trained to teach their standard tenets and methods of information dissemination, so you can expect to receive uniform information from Evidence Based Birth classes. These classes are offered in a variety of durations, from six weeks of online videos to four weeks of one-hour virtual instruction in small groups. The majority of these courses combine online and pre-recorded instruction. Accelerated versions are available and include adjunct videos and reading materials. The classes and virtual contents covering a multitude of pregnancy- and postpartum-related topics are accessible electronically. The major goal of Evidence Based Birth is not advocating for or against the use of medications or methods of pain control, but to provide the information you need to make the most informed decisions at every juncture of your pregnancy journey through labor and birth.

Birthing From Within was established in the late 1990s after a midwife, Pam England, mulled over understanding what modern people need to know about how to give birth in a culture that medicalizes birth. The educators of this class are certified and trained to represent the philosophy of the course. To that end, you can expect individuality from the instructors, including duration, length, and methods of instruction. In large part, the focus of Birthing From Within involves learning to overcome fear, being empowered and in tune with yourself as a birthing individual, and increasing confidence to decrease the likelihood of being vulnerable to birth trauma. Birthing From Within courses are helpful for individuals and those who are partnered. The classes use books, videos, and various methods to bring ceremony and ritual to the labor and birthing process.

BRAXTON-HICKS CONTRACTIONS

Braxton-Hicks (BH) contractions are called "false labor" because they mean that although you are having contractions, labor has not yet begun. In the weeks and days leading up to labor, some may experience increased episodes of cramps, abdominal tightening, or back pain. Early labor can also commonly consist of some forms of cramping or back pain as well. One key difference between this third trimester discomfort and early labor is that one goes away with common remedies. Cramps, contractions, or back pain associated with real labor will not go away despite trying relieving therapies. In the third trimester, BH contractions can be subtle and easy to ignore, or intense and last several hours. To determine whether your contractions are BH, try several things to see if they go away. Have a small snack, drink about 64 ounces of water over the course of an hour, take a shower, lie down to rest, or try some distracting activities such as watching a movie. Real labor contractions will not go away despite anything you try. Labor contractions may also be associated with other changes, such as an increase in vaginal secretions, loss of your mucus plug, leaking of fluid, or some loose stool. It is never wrong to reach out to your pregnancy care provider if you are having contractions and you are concerned about whether they are related to labor.

Chapter 5

During Childbirth

This chapter provides details about the different aspects of your birth plan, including the atmosphere and environment of your labor and birth space, options if an induction becomes necessary, plans for pain management, approaches to medical interventions, and options for the third stage of labor. Although unanticipated emergencies are not very common, I go through ways to manage such events. Your birth plan walks through what will happen during your labor and birth in a sequential method, but understand that everything may not evolve in the progressive way you might have imagined. However, as your labor develops, referring to your preferences for that particular portion of your labor will draw the pathway back to what you had envisioned as your birth goals and will serve as a tool to keep things going in the trajectory that you have planned for.

The terminology you see in the upcoming section will match how the birth plan is arranged. As you develop your own birth plan, I suggest you refer back to this section to refresh your thoughts, inform yourself, and formulate questions you find relevant. You may want to highlight areas that spark reflection and come back to them later with your intended support persons or your provider.

BIRTH STORY: A PLAN OF ACTION

Hialeah had officially penned her birth plan about two days before her son was born, but she had been talking with her partner about the type of birth she wanted for many weeks. When it came to thinking through her preferences, she essentially wrote out what she had envisioned as important to her, paying close attention to her underlying goals of never wanting to be separated from her partner, being involved in all decision making about her care, and having skin-to-skin time with her baby immediately following birth. On the day I saw her for her prenatal appointment, Hialeah was nearing her due date, but we both expected to see each other for the following week's visit. Instead, Hialeah's water broke days later without any signs of labor on the horizon. Although she was admitted to the hospital, she was not in labor and didn't think her birth plan would take effect. Hialeah did anticipate starting penicillin during labor because she had tested positive for a Group B streptococcus (GBS) infection during her second and third trimesters." GBS is an asymptomatic bacteria found in the vagina and rectum that can slightly increase the risk of infection in babies born of GBS-positive mothers.

However, once she discovered meconium in her amniotic fluid when her water broke, the birth plan was immediately put in place. On occasion, when a pregnant individual gets near or past their due date, the baby, practicing new bodily functions, has their first bowel movement. We call this bowel movement meconium. Other times, meconium in the amniotic fluid could mean that the baby has had a period of stress. It is not always clear why the bowel movement occurred, or even when it occurred. When we see meconium in the amniotic fluid of people who are not yet in labor, the discussion becomes whether to administer medication to induce labor or wait to see if labor starts on its own.

Hialeah's labor was induced. Over the next couple of hours while waiting to begin the induction, her baby began to show signs that the meconium wasn't just the regular "I am just showing off that I know how to make poo." The fetal monitor indicated that the baby was having a stressful time inside. Hialeah never was able to start the induction process because adding more stress to a baby already showing signs of stress is generally not a good idea. Instead, we decided to continue to monitor the baby to see if the information on the fetal monitor showed signs of improvement so we could begin the induction. It was only after Hialeah developed a fever that the baby went from sometimes having periods of stress to really having a hard time.

Hialeah's birth plan skipped completely through all the plans she had made for labor and went right to the part of what to do if a situation developed that would necessitate a cesarean birth. This unexpected situation developed fairly rapidly. Although a surgical birth was not what Hialeah had wanted, her birth plan outlined her choices for all possible outcomes.

On Arrival

It is imperative that your team is in alignment with your expectations to ensure a smooth transition from your home to the birth space. This is particularly important if you are meeting some of these people for the first time. Ensure that the team is aware that you have preferences about your care by way of a birth plan. Your birth plan can be provided to your care providers by you, or by a designated member of your birth team who has accompanied you to your birth space. Labor is not an emergency, but when people move quickly, it can feel that way.

If your birth plan is handed over to someone you are meeting for the first time, use this as an opportunity to slow down, reflect on, and reinforce what you are looking to accomplish. Your chosen birth location will dictate many details about what occurs when you first arrive if you have not stated a preference. It is important that the members of your care team acknowledge your well-thought-out plans.

Atmosphere

Think about the options that make you most physically comfortable. Would you prefer to limit the number of guests in your space or does your plan include an expanded support team? If you are laboring outside your home, are there any focal points you would like to see? Now consider the sounds you would like to hear. Is it quiet or do you hear music or some other sounds? Were you hoping to incorporate a soothing scent or aromatherapy into your labor space? Think about how you want the room to feel when you open your eyes. Would you prefer lighting that illuminates your surroundings or a dimmer or natural light? Setting your ideal atmosphere helps your body perform the primal act of labor.

STARTING POSITION

When it is reasonable to do so, early labor should occur at home. If you are not planning on birthing in your home, the ideal is to arrive to your birth space when you are in active labor. During this time, activities you use to cope with labor will not eliminate pain but will help you deal with discomfort. Instinctively, you may find that you get up and move. This is exactly what you want to be doing! As you are moving your body in all its normal ways to manage contractions, your baby is also navigating through their own movements and working with you to facilitate labor.

Standing up

When you feel like you want to stand up, stand up! Get out of the bed. Your body is intuitive and responds to the pressure of your baby's head being applied to your cervix from the inside. Gravity is your friend.

Lying down

Labor is hard work. When you feel like lying down or resting your body, do it. In the most physically taxing moments of labor, there is some time between contractions when your body can benefit from a break from having to support your standing body.

Walking around

Your pelvic bones are a series of bones held together largely by cartilage with hinge-like movements. When you walk, you are moving these joints, and the movements work in synchronicity with your baby to negotiate the optimal position in the pelvis.

Using the shower

Water has long been used for pain management in labor. A benefit of using the shower is to focus the stream on areas where you experience contractions with more intensity.

Submerging in the bathtub

Hydrotherapy in the form of water submersion is a powerful method to manage pain for many individuals throughout all phases of active labor and birth. Weightlessness in water also allows your body to relax between contractions.

WHO'S IN THE ROOM?

Childbirth can be chaotic if you have not established who you would like to have in your birth space. It is wise to be explicit about who can and cannot be in your space and for which portions of your labor. As a rule, your labor is not a spectator sport. Your birth place may commonly use residents, medical students, midwifery students, and others who are present in a learning capacity. You are under no obligation to have any learners at your birth in any capacity if you are uncomfortable with their presence. The same principle goes for requests from family members or friends who feel it is important to be at the birth. Ultimately, this is your birth, and you get to decide who you want to participate and in which ways.

WHAT'S IN THE ROOM?

The place where you birth is likely equipped with various options to aid you throughout your labor. Better to have tools available for you to use in labor than to need a tool and not have it. People commonly try several methods of pain management before finding ones that work best. Others find one method that works well, and use only that tool throughout their labor. Whether this is your first labor or your tenth, you won't know what will work best for you until you try it.

Bean bag chair

These bags allow your body to sink into a weightless support, which is particularly helpful between contractions to recharge.

Birthing ball

When used in labor, large exercise balls, yoga balls, and peanut balls transform into powerful tools. You can sit or rock on them, lie against them, or use one between your knees. Keeping your pelvis open and mobile is the goal.

Birthing bed

Hospital beds can be transformed in various ways to help you hang, lean, pull, push, squat, or swing with the support of the bed.

Birthing pool, shower, or tub

Hydrotherapy in a pool, shower, or tub helps with pain control during labor and birth, shortens the first stage, and decreases the need for epidural use.

Birthing stool

These stools are very low to the ground and emulate a squat, widening your pelvis. Some people labor on the stool, while others find the squatting position on the stool to be helpful for pushing and even delivering their babies.

Squatting bar

The squatting bar is an attachment to the bed and, like the birthing stool, provides a way for the body to get into the squatting position. Additionally, the bar can be used to dangle from or as leverage and traction during the pushing phase.

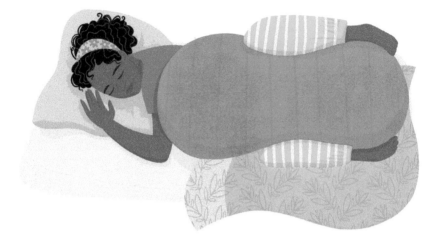

The pain of labor is distinct from the pain caused by a pathologic process. Labor pain comes with a normal, human purpose. It has a beginning and a definitive end. You will spend hours, potentially days, in the same location for labor, birth, and recovery. The physical space and all the ways you find comfort through this process are so important. Setting your intentions to find methods to bring yourself whatever semblance of comfort you can are essential to creating and implementing a successful birth plan through a process that is undeniably painful.

Soft lights and stillness

Certain methods of labor coping skills, such as HypnoBirthing, require a specific absence of external stimuli. The type of lighting, the amount and type of noise, and even how others move in and about your birth space are options to consider. Some birth spaces have a mood that conveys highly intense energy, which may look like brighter lights, audible music, and background conversations.

Other spaces will convey a quieter, more serene atmosphere and may have diffused lighting, ambient noises, and only quiet whispers. Having options and tools to be able to pivot between these moods is something to consider. For out-of-home births, items brought in to the birth space should be cleared for use in the space, particularly open candle flames or lighting that must be plugged in.

Music and aromatherapy

Music can have an important impact on how your body feels. Remembering that you want to facilitate a calm and relaxed body whenever possible, consider adding music to your labor environment if you find you have a relationship with music that accomplishes that for you. Many people find aromatherapy has non-medicinal benefits to alleviate fear, anxiety, pain, and tension. In my experience, aromatherapy works particularly well in labor if you have had success with using aromatherapy to alleviate similar symptoms in the past. If aroma therapy is something you want to consider, include it in your birth plan. For out-of-home births, remember to clear essential oils for those who may have allergies or sensitivities.

Interruptions and exams

When someone is doing really well using their coping strategies to get themselves through contraction after contraction, I call this "getting in the groove." This groove can last for a few contractions or sometimes for hours. When the groove is interrupted, it can be difficult to return to effective coping. In active labor, and particularly in transition, you can throw someone off their groove by interrupting them to ask non-pertinent questions or perform a cervical exam. It is impossible to predict when you will get into a groove during your labor, or to predict when you'll need time to refocus and restore. For this reason, many people prefer to limit the use of vaginal exams and interruptions unless truly necessary.

Clothing

For individuals not birthing at home or at a birth center, consider what you'll wear during labor and postpartum recovery. You will be provided a hospital gown that opens in the back as the standard get-up when you arrive in labor. For some, this option means one less piece of laundry they have to do. For others, the standard hospital gown disrupts their ability to be as comfortable as they could be. For this reason, if you prefer to labor in something other than what is provided, include the clothing in your plan.

Food and drink

Childbirth is exhausting, and many people choose to eat and drink energy-rich foods and drinks throughout this process. A wide variety of options are available to support hydration as the body works extremely hard. For those not laboring at home or at a birth center, investigate the available options. Some labor units do not restrict eating, whereas others do. Those who desire an epidural for pain control should be prepared to manage the duration of their labor with limited volumes of clear beverages. The hospital will have standard options, so plan accordingly.

Labor Preferences

For the most part, your labor preferences will make up the most detailed part of your birth plan. These preferences cover everything from inductions to pain management to how you and your baby are monitored throughout the labor and birth process. Since there are so many options to consider, and so many possible divergences, a well-thought-out birth plan considers ways that labor commonly changes course. Once again, I suggest visualizing the end point of your labor and working backward. The choices for all sections of your birth plan should try to reinforce and support your labor and birth goals.

LABOR PREP

Ultimately, we hope your baby comes out of your vagina without much pomp and circumstance. Many people wonder if there is anything they should be doing to prepare their external physical body for labor. Most providers will say no. Overwhelmingly, it makes no difference to your provider whether you choose to have body hair; choosing to ceremoniously groom for labor is your business and literally has nothing to do with anyone else.

INDUCTION

One of the most common events that leads to induction, occurring in 8 percent of pregnancies, is the water breaking but labor not starting. Most commonly, labor begins within 24 hours of a person's water breaking. Ruptured membranes pose an increased risk of infection because the protective barrier is unable to prevent infections that may enter the uterus through the vagina. You and the birthing team will discuss ways to monitor the baby and induce labor. Patients may choose to forgo an immediate induction, opting for labor to start naturally. There are many ways to induce labor, including the use of hormones such as oxytocin. Knowing your options will help you remain calm if your birth plan takes a detour.

Breast stimulation

Stimulation of the nipples and breasts releases pulses of the hormone oxytocin, which causes labor contractions. Massage the breast working your way to the nipples in a gentle, firm, rhythmical fashion. Alternatively, a willing partner can suck on the nipples to stimulate a release of these hormones as well. Another possibility is using a breast pump on a comfortable setting to stimulate hormonal release. Nipple stimulation seems to be most helpful when performed intermittently over the course of a few days.

Walking

When contractions have already started, sometimes walking seems to intensify contractions. Walking is an excellent way in pregnancy to keep the pelvis and hips from laying stagnant, while you increase your cardiovascular activity. If your water has broken, the effect of gravity is accentuated as you walk and you continue to lose water and your baby descends lower into your pelvis. Remember not to overdo it; remain hydrated and rest when needed.

Herbs

Red raspberry leaf or evening primrose can be taken in the last weeks of pregnancy to help soften the cervix in preparation for labor. Other herbs, such as blue cohosh (*Caulophyllum thalictroides*) and black cohosh (*Cimicifuga racemosa*) have been used in regimens to stimulate the uterus to begin labor. Herbs for the purpose of prompting labor contractions should be obtained from a qualified herbalist because of the potential toxic side effects some individuals experience.

Castor oil and enemas

Castor oil will stimulate the bowels in many individuals; for some, this stimulation happens in a particularly aggressive manner. The paralytic effect of castor oil on the GI system seems to also have a side effect of stimulating contractions. For this reason, some look to this ingredient to use in some "midwifery brew" recipes designed to help start or increase contractions. Enemas are another possibility for stimulating the bowels. There is no reason, however, that an enema should be considered a routine preparation for labor.

Chiropractic adjustment

During pregnancy, many hormonal changes loosen and soften ligaments. Chiropractic body adjustments that release a hormone called relaxin—which relaxes ligaments and the soft tissue in the legs, hips, and pelvis—can have a cascading effect and help bring on labor.

Acupuncture

Acupuncture has been used for centuries. This method can alleviate pain in the body, aid the body in restoring its own balance, and prompt labor contractions to begin without medical intervention. Today, licensed acupuncturists are used throughout pregnancy, and later in pregnancy, they can help the cervix begin the ripening process.

Prostaglandins

Prostaglandins are a natural hormonal substance found in the body that have a softening effect on the cervix. Misoprostol is a medication traditionally used to treat ulcers. Used off-label, misoprostol, along with another medication, dinoprostone, are the two chemical prostaglandins that work similarly to produce a ripening of the cervix. These medications can be administered in various ways and in different doses and using different regimens. Due to potential side effects, these substances should be administered only in hospital settings with continuous fetal heart rate monitoring.

Sexual intercourse

It seems like getting into labor has been all about hormones, and it really is. Having sexual intercourse, particularly if you are able to achieve orgasm, releases a wonderful surge of, you guessed it, the main hormone responsible for labor, oxytocin. If you are having vaginal intercourse with a penis, semen is also a wonderful source of natural prostaglandin. If your water has broken and you are waiting for contractions to begin, however, you should avoid putting anything in your vagina thereby preventing bacteria from entering the uterus, where it can cause an infection.

Rupturing membranes

The reason we expect you to go into labor within 24 hours of your water breaking is the accompanying release of hormones that eventually cascade into contractions that stimulate labor. The biggest concern with purposely rupturing your membranes for the purpose of inducing labor is that the longer the membranes have been ruptured, the greater the risk of getting an infection.

For those who need to be treated with antibiotics throughout their labor because of GBS bacteria, purposely breaking this protective barrier prior to labor requires a discussion of the risks versus benefits. Even in the absence of GBS, at any point prior to or during labor, purposely breaking this barrier is worth discussion.

Stripping membranes

The process of stripping the membranes is thought to release hormones that can compel labor contractions to begin. Stripping the membranes involves a provider inserting their fingers through a softened and ripe cervix and separating the bag of water from the edges of the cervix. This manual interruption may also work because it irritates the cervix and lower uterus, causing contractions. In people just on the precipice of spontaneous labor, these induced contractions can stimulate labor. The risks of stripping the membranes are unintended rupture of the membranes and cervical bleeding.

Pitocin

Pitocin is the synthetic version of your body's natural hormone. This medication is excluded for use in out-of-hospital settings because continuous fetal monitoring is required to monitor the duration and frequency of contractions as well as the baby's response to the contractions. The principal risk with use of this medication is tachysystole, or too many contractions without a break. The dose of this medication is administered by IV and is subjectively titrated and monitored by nurses in an attempt to replicate a pattern of contractions with a regular and frequent pattern.

Throughout labor, there are two primary ways to accomplish fetal assessment. Outside of hospitals, the baby's heart rate is monitored by intermittent auscultation as the standard of care. This is accomplished by listening to the baby at specific intervals and times throughout the course of labor with the use of a handheld doppler or fetoscope. The second way to accomplish fetal assessment is by continuous external fetal monitoring (EFM). Some circumstances, such as use of epidural and some medications, as well as pregnancy risk factors will require EFM. This type of monitoring has been shown to increase the risk of cesarean and forceps- or vacuum-assisted deliveries without the value of seeing differences in improvement for babies. The high rate of error in interpreting EFM is a reason low-risk people may choose to opt out of receiving continuous fetal monitoring in hospital settings.

PAIN RELIEF

Many options for medicinal pain relief may not completely eliminate all the pain from labor, so learning about alternative pain management strategies is useful for anyone, regardless of whether they plan to use medicine during labor. Contractions get closer together with increasing intensity and duration until they occur in regular enough frequency to cause the cervix to dilate and efface. In active labor, we see contractions anywhere from two minutes to five minutes from the start of one contraction to the start of the next one, and they can last 45 to 90 seconds. Normal contractions can occur outside these parameters, too. In addition to other signs, pain that consistently does not stop can be pain unrelated to normal labor.

The techniques listed below can be used alone or in combination with other methods of pain relief in labor. Your birth space will determine which options are available for use.

Acupressure and acupuncture

Acupressure uses pressure points to alleviate common symptoms such as pain, nausea, and fatigue. Acupuncture uses similar points to those of acupressure on the body to support pain management. Both methods have shown increased labor satisfaction and can sometimes shorten duration. Acupressure points can be taught to labor support persons with relative ease without risk to the baby or birther, whereas acupuncture is performed by a licensed individual. Check with your birth space whether acupuncturists will be able to treat you while you're admitted.

Patterned breathing techniques

Some labor management techniques, such as Lamaze, emphasize the use of patterned breathing as the primary pain management strategy. Regardless of whether you learned this particular approach, patterned breathing can be effective for labor pain. Shifting focus from the pain of your contractions to intentional, focused, patterned breathing has been shown to decrease anxiety and perception of pain and increase oxygen.

Heat or cold therapy

The uterus is the primary muscular organ responsible for your contractions, and like any other muscle, after several hours of intense working it can become sore. This soreness can be helped with heat or cold therapy. Some liken the intensity of contractions to intense menstrual cramps, so they share similar pain relief methods. For focused pain relief to these areas, applying heat or cold to the area may decrease pain. Heat or cold can also facilitate relaxation.

Water therapy (pool, shower, or tub)

Soaking or showering can increase the relief that heat provides sore muscles. Hydrotherapy through pools, showers, or tubs is widely available, even in hospital settings. Buoyancy and the ability to use streams of water to focus on particular areas are some reasons people find water to be a particularly effective pain control measure.

Demerol, narcotics, sedatives, or tranquilizers

Demerol, narcotics, sedatives, and tranquilizers taken in labor are typically reserved for hospital birth and are administered by injection into the muscle or by IV. These interventions are not commonly a first line for pain control for several reasons. Primarily, there is concern that the medications are absorbed into your circulation, and the effects can be seen in the baby for those who are on continuous fetal monitoring. Additionally, narcotics can have lingering effects on the baby after they are born that interfere with their alertness, feeding, or respiratory effort. The use of narcotics, sedatives, or tranquilizers are not ideal for those who are in active labor, or who may birth soon, but these medications are most commonly administered when the birth is still a long way away.

Distraction

Our brains make it difficult to give our total concentration to several things at one time. For this reason, distraction with other activities is an effective tool in early labor as one transitions into more active labor and contractions take on a quality and intensity that take over the primary senses. Distraction tends to be less effective as a solitary tool. However, distraction is a key factor as you implement other tools to manage and tolerate labor. Anything you do to cope with labor is really just a specific type of distraction.

Vocalizations

Labor contractions are repetitive, so coping mechanisms must also be employed with repetition to be effective. Chanting, grunting, humming, moaning, or singing in sync with contractions can be a successful strategy. Contractions start out mildly, building with intensity until they reach their peak. The contraction then recedes in the same fashion, tapering off in intensity just as it increased and decreased for the previous contraction. Those who use vocalizations typically mirror their contractions.

Hypnosis, meditation, or deep (or guided) relaxation

Relaxation is a major focus of many prenatal education courses. Classes such as HypnoBirthing use structured techniques to facilitate a hypnotic-like awareness to reduce the perception of pain. This strategy works to replace tension, fear, and physical manifestations of pain with pleasant sensations, calming sounds, favorable sights, and intentional thoughts. These methods can be helpful if you have someone else guide you through the relaxation or meditation exercises, or if you choose to lead yourself through exercises on your own.

Aromatherapy, massage, or reflexology

Essential oils used for massage or alone in a diffuser may provide benefits of aromatherapy. Massage does not need to be of professional grade to be helpful for pain relief or to promote relaxation in labor. Reflexology is done by applying pressure to pressure points to relieve pain and other symptoms during labor. Practitioners of this method are reflexologists, but just as non-specialists can perform massage, individuals who are not reflexologists can be taught where the pressure points are to use in labor.

Standard epidural

Epidural anesthesia is the most common form of pain control in the United States. Epidurals are narcotics administered in a continuous dose through the intrathecal route, or the thin layer of tissue surrounding the spinal cord, after a local numbing agent is given. In most instances, pain relief improves over the course of 20 minutes and additional doses of medication can be self-administered as needed through a patient-controlled button. Unlike with the use of IV or intramuscular narcotics administered through an injection into the muscle, intrathecal narcotics don't typically produce the side effects of nausea or lethargy, and we don't normally see changes in the EFM that would indicate evidence of the narcotic in fetal circulation. Ideally, the standard dose of medication in an epidural will not make you completely numb; the bottom half of your body will have markedly decreased sensation without a paralyzing effect. In working epidurals, contraction pain is considerably decreased while allowing you to still be aware of the sensation of pressure. Individual reactions and bodily functions following an epidural will vary based on many individual factors.

Walking epidural

A standard epidural changes the way your lower body reacts to stimuli; a walking epidural, however, allows the ability to walk and perform biologic functions such as urinating. The unpredictability of the individual responses to the medications in the epidural are reasons there may be some reluctance on the part of anesthesiologists or nurse anesthetists to administer the epidural using this method.

TENS machine

A TENS unit provides electrical impulses through small adhesive probes applied to the skin in areas where pain is experienced. This method is thought to work because of how the perception of pain requires a sensation to be transmitted along nerve routes as the pain signal is sent to your brain. The TENS machine uses electrical impulses to interrupt the pain pathways, so the message that you are having pain is interrupted.

Nitrous oxide

The use of inhaled nitrous oxide (N_2O) gas is the most commonly used form of medicinal pain control in many countries outside the United States. The N_2O is mixed with oxygen and is self-administered through a technique that limits the gas from escaping into the air. Nitrous oxide gas is only available from licensed healthcare providers, and many hospitals, birth centers, and home birth practices have it available. N_2O can be administered throughout any portion of labor and birth, and it can be used during laceration repair. The gas is inhaled through a mask that covers your mouth and nose. It works within a few inhalations, and the effects wear off within a few breaths after the mask has been removed from your face. The biggest reported side effects are nausea or vomiting, dizziness, lightheadedness, and claustrophobia.

KEY ADVICE: GETTING HELP WITH PAIN

When it boils down to it, there are two major keys about pain and labor: Pain should be manageable and tolerable. If the pain can no longer be tolerated, or if you are no longer able to manage the pain, human nature compels you to do something about it. Fortunately, in labor, you can do many things about the pain. Pain management is about the preparation you put into it, the availability of management options, and the ability to use your learned strategies when the time comes. When you, as the birthing person, have agency and autonomy over your body as well as education and can prepare, labor pain is manageable and tolerable. You should plan to use a combination of methods, as the most manageable and tolerable labor experiences include using a variety of techniques throughout the course of labor and birth to cope with discomfort and pain. Understanding methods of coping, including your options for managing the pain, can be a critical factor in having a satisfactory birth experience.

Many people pivot from what they thought would make their birth experience manageable and tolerable because their strategy was not working. When people understand which pain management options are available, they typically will ask for medicinal approaches if they desire them. Each labor is different. Try not to box yourself into the idea that only one particular strategy will work for you, and be open to being flexible for what works in the moment, knowing what options are available in your chosen birth space.

A practice that has fallen out of routine use and is only performed in emergency situations is the episiotomy. This intervention uses scissors to make a cut in the perineum to allow for soft tissue reduction just as the baby is crowning. This cut is done in situations when it has been determined that the skin or tissue on the perineum is slowing down the birth. Episiotomy can also make space to accommodate the application of forceps or a vacuum, or to make space for hands in the rare occurrence that a baby needs physical assistance to be delivered.

DELIVERY PREFERENCES

The time between the last contraction to the birth of the baby can be moments, so without some forethought or planning, you can miss an opportunity to relay what your preferences are for these first few moments of your baby's external life. Nearly all birth spaces now routinely follow practices that facilitate your baby's smooth transition to extrauterine life. These can include immediate skin-to-skin contact, allowing the cord to cease pulsations before cutting, and even rooming-in. If you have strong preferences, clear communication about what you'd like prior to the birth of your baby works best.

Position

For pushing, find the position that feels right for you unless the use of epidural anesthesia or other medications limit your movement or ability to support one's own body weight. Otherwise, squat bars, foot pedals, bed leg supports, and stirrups can be used for support and traction for births that occur on a bed. Sitting, squatting, leaning, standing, and side-lying are all reasonable positions, and movement into assorted positions for pushing can help the baby navigate through the narrowest parts of the pelvis.

Sights and sounds

Visualizing what happens when you push can serve as motivation as the delivery becomes imminent. Some people choose to see this process by requesting a mirror to watch as the head emerges from their body. Many also choose to welcome the baby with music or calm sounds. As the baby makes its appearance, a positive sensory experience may be a calming tool for you and your baby.

Pushing and catching

It's important to know what to expect during the pushing phase of delivery. Pushing occurs during a contraction, not the period of rest between contractions. Without awareness of when contractions are occurring, self-directed pushing might be impossible. For that reason, some may benefit from some instructions with how to coordinate their bearing efforts.

Epidurals can suppress the natural reactions of the body, sometimes concealing the start of the second stage of labor. Some may experience an increase in the amount of vaginal or rectal pressure, or instead of feeling intermittent pressure, might feel a more constant pressure. A cervical exam, among other signs, will tell if the cervix has dilated to 10 centimeters and it is time to push. The loss of sensation with the use of an epidural can make it difficult to coordinate what you feel with what your body is doing.

For those laboring without an epidural, the beginning of second stage labor may be covert or clear as day. Pushing is most effective when the individual pushes when, how, and for how long they feel like pushing. When the body is left to labor on its own, pushing is an instinctual process very similar to vomiting. You won't need much help identifying when it comes time to push; your body will just do it. The same goes for the actual catching process, which can happen pretty quickly regardless of how long someone has been pushing. Those who have caught many babies have a general rule: Don't drop the baby! That being said, the babies are slippery and wet when they come out, so if you think you may want someone other than your provider to catch your baby, it's often a good idea to let this preference be known ahead of time so the catching process goes smoothly.

Breech birth

Babies can be born facing practically any direction. A baby is considered breech when their feet, knees, or bottom are poised to emerge from the vagina first instead of the head. There are several ways to manage this situation. In some instances, when a baby settles into a breech position, providers will offer breech deliveries and will catch the baby in whatever position they come out. Your provider may offer you an external cephalic version, a procedure used to manually move the baby into a head-down position. Other providers may suggest a combination of acupressure or moxibustion (a therapy from traditional Chinese medicine that involves burning dried mugwort) to help babies rotate. Many people have also reported success with babies moving into a head-down position with use of a specific exercise technique called *spinning babies*. Although babies can come out in almost any direction, they cannot come out in every position (for example, sideways). In some instances, after all the options have been considered for the safest birth, a surgical birth may be the recommendation.

A forceps is an instrument composed of two metal pieces, similar to salad tongs, that encompass the head of the baby. A vacuum is applied to the top of the baby's head and both suction and traction are used to guide the baby's head through delivery.

A vacuum or forceps-assisted vaginal delivery is attempted when the birth of the baby is imminent but needs to be expedited. These methods support a vaginal delivery once the baby's head has descended low enough into the pelvis to be safely helped through the vagina.

CESAREAN

The majority of first-time cesarean births are not planned. There are three main reasons for a cesarean birth once you have already started labor: the cervix stops dilating, the baby does not descend low enough into the pelvis to achieve a vaginal birth, or there is an emergency that makes it unsafe to keep your baby inside any longer. Largely, cesarean births are not an emergency and there is time to administer a type of spinal anesthesia very similar to an epidural for those who did not labor with one. For those who have had an epidural, a different type of medication is administered through the catheter in place. This stronger medication brings the epidural to a level of anesthesia that is high enough to permit surgery. The goal in most surgical births, even in certain emergencies, is to use the type of anesthesia that keeps the birther as awake and alert as possible for the birth of their baby.

Whether a birth occurs urgently, or if it has been under consideration for several hours, you still have options. In the United States, approximately one in three hospital births will result in a surgical birth, and non-hospital settings will see a surgical birth 1 in 16 times. Not planning for this type of birth limits your ability to decide if the standard of care is something you want and would agree to after knowing all your options. Who would you like to accompany you? How much or how little of the surgery do you want to see? What would you like to do regarding decisions about the cord detachment and placenta? Would you like skin-to-skin contact for you or your support person in the operating room? If the baby needs to be separated from you, what is the plan for your support person? Will they go with the baby or stay with you in the operating room? Your postpartum recovery will change as well, with two to three days expected for a typical recovery in the hospital, whereas people who had vaginal deliveries are usually discharged after one or two days.

KEY ADVICE: HEALING AFTER A CESAREAN SECTION

Very few people begin their birth plan with a cesarean in mind. I would encourage you not to consider this option as an afterthought. A surgical birth is a possibility for anyone having a baby. The way your pregnancy or labor unfolds, where you decide to have your baby, who you decide to have as your provider, what you choose for pain control, and many other decisions and events throughout pregnancy and labor will either increase or decrease your risk for a cesarean section. Some, after an unplanned cesarean birth, have perceived their birth process as a failure, but that is simply unfounded. Vaginal births are one of only two ways your baby can be born. Start by appreciating the value of planning for both eventualities in your birth plan. Care and consideration for your preferences will give you a head start for any emotional healing that will need to happen while you are physically healing from a cesarean birth.

Unless you have a scheduled cesarean section, proceeding with a surgical birth will accompany many emotions. Disappointment, shame, or anger at the inability to delivery vaginally can take longer to recover from than the physical aspects of surgery. These negative feelings can be compounded if your preferences were not elicited, or you didn't know that you had any options through this process. In the time after an unplanned surgical birth, some may find themselves replaying their birth scenarios, looking to place blame or change circumstances. When people are having trouble reconciling the complicated layers of disappointment surrounding their birth, I would encourage them to reach out to their support person, doula, or provider for ways to process the outcome of your birth. Fortunately, one cesarean birth does not mean that future births will follow the same path. The safest method for many people who have had a cesarean section is a trial of labor, which has made vaginal birth after a cesarean (VBAC) a common practice. Your options to be supported through a VBAC will depend largely on your chosen birth place and provider.

THIRD STAGE LABOR

Finally! The baby is out! Particular attention should be paid to this period of time because it happens very quickly. When the baby comes out and takes their first breaths of air, dynamic shifts are occurring in your baby's circulation. They are moving from reliance on the placenta to their own little heart. During these incredible moments, the umbilical cord, once pulsating powerfully at 110 to 160 times a minute, begins to slow down. As the baby takes over its own circulation, the changes in the pumping of blood can be felt in the umbilical cord, starting with a bounding pulse before slowing and eventually stopping. This signals that all the blood your baby needs has now shifted away from the placenta, which has finally completed its job, and to the baby.

The umbilical cord might pulse for less than 60 seconds up to several minutes following the baby's birth. Letting the cord cease pulsation on its own improves the baby's red blood cell volume, decreases the risk for the necessity of blood transfusions, and decreases some of the risks of gastrointestinal and bleeding complications, commonly seen in preterm infants. For this reason, the common practice is to leave the cord intact at least until the period of pulsations has ended. Some may choose to cut the umbilical cord themselves after it has emptied, or they may designate another person to cut the cord after the placenta has been delivered. Still others will not cut the cord at all, allowing for a natural separation, as seen in lotus births. For those collecting stem cells, the efficacy, quality, and ability to bank cord blood relies on being able to harvest a minimum volume of blood from the umbilical cord when it is still full, before it stops pulsating. Your decision about the use of the placenta or how to treat the umbilical cord must be made well in advance of delivery.

What happens immediately following the birth of your baby also depends on the practices of your provider and chosen birth place. One of the jobs of your uterus after the placenta comes out is to begin the work of getting back to its pre-pregnant size. If the uterus isn't squeezing and contracting down, bleeding will increase. Providers may administer pitocin to try and prevent a postpartum hemorrhage, while others will not administer this medication unless there is more than a normal amount of bleeding, and after other methods of controlling bleeding have been used. Choosing to accept pitocin in the third stage of labor as a preventive measure should be clearly indicated on your birth plan.

Chapter 6

After Childbirth

This chapter provides information about what happens in the moments, hours, and days following your baby's birth. You'll also review options related to situations in which the baby is separated from you, such as delaying any tests until you're present.

You will read through the timing expectation for medical tests, medication administration, feeding your baby, rest and recovery, and will examine whether circumcision applies to you. A clearly defined birth plan, your chosen birth location, and your provider will help you define your options.

BIRTH STORY: WHAT'S BEST FOR BABY

Ivy was a first-time mom who was unsure about what she wanted to happen immediately after childbirth. She was certain of many of the choices she had made, including the use of an epidural for pain control. The majority of people have a pretty good idea about the care they would like to receive once they have been educated on their options. Areas of labor or birth where people lack information or are fearful generally take the most time to figure out for the birth plan. By 41 weeks, Ivy still wasn't sure how she felt about having her baby skin to skin immediately after birth. Would she be covered in blood or fluids? Would she prefer to have the benefits of immediate skin-to-skin contact, followed by a golden hour, that would keep her baby in contact with her after birth? Or would she feel more comfortable having the baby cleaned off and wrapped up as she held her?

When contemplating these decisions, again I encourage people to work backward. I asked Ivy to see herself pushing the baby out and the midwife catching the baby. Where did she see the baby being placed? Ivy reported that she saw a towel on her chest, the baby placed atop the towel, dried off. Her lingering question was whether she would feel okay about having a wet, possibly bloody, baby being placed on her skin? Labor and childbirth are in fact filled with several deeply personal decisions that can feel monumental. Keep in mind, birth is very rarely an emergency, so when critical decisions must be made, there is normally time to confer with the laboring person. When the baby comes out, it takes minimal effort for the provider to ask where you would like them to place the baby, and barely any effort for your nurse or other labor support person to either place a towel across your chest, or to remove a towel from your chest. The keys in these scenarios are preparation and communication.

The provider needs to know that you would like to be asked in that moment and your support person will also need to be prepared to help you achieve your goals. With a proper birth plan, you can absolutely be provided care in alignment with your needs.

Ultimately, Ivy's labor plans went according to what she wanted. To her, the unpredictability of labor felt like a setback because her second stage lasted four hours. She was exhausted and elated by the time her daughter finally made her way out, offering a loud and robust cry. After pushing for so long, Ivy might not have even recalled that this moment had been important to her. Her midwife was aware, though, that Ivy wanted to decide how her daughter should be taken care of. After so much work, Ivy decided that though she was not as scared of fluids, she still wanted to have her daughter dried off and placed on a towel. Ivy was shown respect and autonomy about what she wanted, and her birth plan was simply a tool that helped her accomplish her goals.

Newborn Procedures

Like the women you have read about here, you will have a unique story. Some parts of your labor will be remembered in great detail, whereas others might feel like a blur. In whatever way your labor unfolds, it will eventually come to a close when you hold your baby, whom you have worked so hard for. In this moment, for many the focus and attention shifts to the baby, as they take in the smallest details of this whole perfect human who has come from their body. This portion of the birth plan will remind you that birth is not an emergency, and even when you are distracted, having an outline in place will help you see what you want to happen immediately after birth.

SKIN-TO-SKIN CONTACT

Skin-to-skin contact means that the baby is held directly against their parent's skin. The benefits of this practice include improved breastfeeding, bonding, baby temperature regulation, and glucose control. Many studies also show that mothers reported improved satisfaction with their birth experience following skin-to-skin contact. These benefits are seen in the immediate window after birth and even later for those who continue this practice throughout the postpartum period. Like Ivy, you will have to decide if you want immediate skin-to-skin contact, or if you prefer to wait until later. For those having a surgical birth, preparations for this contact will require some additional considerations because of the position needed for surgery, and some assistance in securing the baby. Other considerations will be whether and when you would prefer to bathe the baby. Bathing the baby before the first 24 hours can disrupt the vernix, or protective coating on their skin, from naturally absorbing, which is why some parents delay the first bath.

PROCEDURE PROTOCOL

This section of the birth plan will give direction in case of a medical emergency. In situations where the baby is separated from you, will you prefer to have your support person remain with you, or would you like to have them accompany the baby? You will also make decisions about how your baby is to be fed in the instance of prolonged separation, and whether any procedures or tests be delayed until they can be done in your presence.

MEDICAL TESTS AND INTERVENTIONS

This small section covers various tests and interventions that may occur after birth. Many of these procedures are common, some are non-medically indicated, while others, depending on where you live, may even be state mandated. You should know what these tests and medications are for should you plan for anything outside of what is typically offered.

Eye drops and ointments

As a preventive measure for serious eye infection in the baby, erythromycin administration will be offered after birth. Some choose to delay application of this ointment until after the golden hour and breastfeeding, so it will not interfere with bonding.

Vitamin K

A rare, but life-threating, situation known as vitamin K deficiency bleeding (VKDB) results from severe lack of vitamin K and causes bleeding in the brains of babies. As a preventive measure, pediatricians recommend a one-time shot of vitamin K given in the muscle of babies to prevent a certain type of VKDB, particularly in breastfed babies because of the low levels of vitamin K found in breast milk. Those choosing this injection may opt to delay it until after the golden hour. In other countries, oral doses of vitamin K are used, so some people choose to use an oral regimen instead. The variations in the oral dosages, the availability of the oral medication, and the efficacy of oral preparations are reasons many pediatricians recommend the injection over the oral preparation.

Vaccines

Vaccines are a controversial topic, yet the very first time you will have to make a decision on whether to have your child vaccinated may very well be shortly after their birth. The hepatitis B vaccine may be offered anywhere from the time of birth to just prior to discharge from the hospital, with some parents choosing to delay this vaccination until the first pediatrician visit. Your plans for how you would like to approach vaccines, along with any variations in the recommended scheduling, should be discussed well ahead of time with your chosen pediatrician.

PKU testing

About 24 hours following birth, a series of screening tests will be offered. Many states mandate these tests. Some call this a phenylketonuria (PKU) test. PKU is actually a rare inherited disorder and not only the test name. This collection of a few drops of blood obtained through a heel prick of your baby will check for PKU, as well as a minimum of 34 metabolic and hereditary disorders. The rationale for testing in a particular window of time has to do with the ability of the test to pick up disorders that would otherwise not register unless a life-threatening situation were to occur. Depending on your location, it would be highly unusual for these tests to be offered immediately in the labor and birth spaces; they would instead take place within days following the birth. Knowing which tests will be offered, as well as the timeline for collection of the blood samples, are preferences to indicate on your birth plan.

Hearing test

Newborn hearing tests are state mandated because early detection of hearing loss is critical to learning, language, and brain development. In hospital birth spaces and many birth centers, this screening test is administered prior to discharge, but pediatricians with the appropriate equipment can also perform it in their office. The test is quick and painless and can be done while the baby is quiet and calm by placing a soft earphone into the baby's ear canal. When a sound is made, a measurement of the brain response and the echo of the sound against the ear drum is evaluated. Your preferences may include when and where you would like this testing done.

Circumcision is the removal of the foreskin that covers the penis. This skin is removed for religious, cultural, or personal reasons. Whether to circumcise your baby's penis is a highly debated topic because there is no medical reason to prophylactically perform this procedure. When parents choose to circumcise while in the hospital, it usually is done within a day or two following birth with the use of local anesthetics. And those who are having circumcisions done for religious reasons may have the procedure done several days following discharge from the birth space. Having a circumcision in the hospital allows time for parents to learn to care for the area of skin that has been cut, as well as to be educated on signs that might indicate a problem. Your preferences for whether or when you plan on having your baby circumcised are important to put on your birth plan.

BREASTFEEDING OR CHEST-FEEDING

Human milk is the ideal food for newborn human babies. The short- and long-term benefits have been extensively studied. A few benefits for exclusively breast milk–fed infants include decreased episodes of upper respiratory illnesses, ear infections, and diaper rashes, and decreased incidents of diabetes and asthma later in life. For those who are choosing to breastfeed, it is not uncommon to need assistance with learning this new skill, especially for those who have undergone a surgical birth or have issues related to the structure of their anatomy, such as having had breast surgery or inverted or flat nipples, or related to the structure of the baby's anatomy, such as a tongue- or lip-tie, or short latch.

Of utmost consideration is the case of experiencing an unexpected prolonged separation of the baby from its intended food source. Water substitution in a baby younger than six months may put infants at risk for serious and life-threatening complications. You should consider beforehand what your plans would be for formula substitution in the event of a prolonged separation or in the event of medical reason.

There are also situations where human milk stops being the best option to feed your baby. Even in cases where breastfeeding is not possible or feasible, lactation specialists are skilled in developing strategies for continuing to provide breast milk through pumping and other milk removal methods. Formula substitutions may be the most medically feasible option for some infants.

Rest and Recovery

The final part of the birth plan concerns rest and recovery. Your baby has finally had their first feed, you have accomplished all your immediate birth plan goals, and you are now taking in the first few hours of your new role. Your baby, whom you have come to know so well as an inhabitant and constant companion for the past several months, has arrived, marking a celebratory beginning of this new life as is evidenced by the work your body was able to accomplish. This part of the journey does not stop here. The next several days and weeks of your initial recovery will be laid out in your preferences to continue to guide your support team, friends, and family, who are likely very excited for your baby's arrival. Your pre-arranged preferences for these people give them the

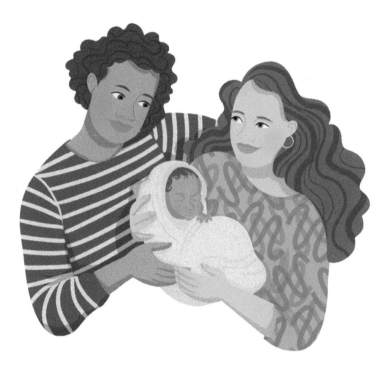

benefit of knowing exactly what you expect during this important time period. Your newly postpartum course requires just as
much care and consideration as your pregnancy, labor, and birth
journey have. Your preferences for this time should not be looked
at as an afterthought.

ROOMING-IN

Several decades ago, in a push to improve breastfeeding, the
World Health Organization and UNICEF launched a program
that included specific action steps hospitals could take to help
promote, support, and advocate for breastfeeding. Hospitals that
have formally initiated these steps are designated *baby friendly*
facilities in which a nursery is not available. For the purpose of
care and observation of the infant for periods of time, parents
are encouraged to room-in with their babies 24-7. Hospitals
not designated as *baby friendly* may mean a nursery is available

on-site for the purpose of new parents choosing not to utilize 24-hour rooming-in with their baby, and instead opting to use the nurse-staffed nursery for periods of rest after a particularly long or arduous labor or birth. Studies have returned mixed results on the benefits of rooming-in on breastfeeding success, but the positive effects of increased confidence and bonding are the main reasons parents choose the room-in option during their hospital stay.

VISITORS

Loved ones will be excited to hear about the arrival of your baby, and some will want to hear your story. Many people may just assume you are accepting visitors into your birth space as you begin your initial postpartum recovery course. Whatever your birth space, the early recovery may include an assortment of feelings. While likely very joyous, the next several hours and days may include periods when you are physically uncomfortable and exhausted, or even emotionally overwhelmed. If you think you would prefer to forgo most, some, or all visitors during this time, this decision is entirely up to you. You know your family and friends best, so if you find that you need to set these boundaries beforehand, it may be wise to address them in discussion prior to labor to avoid surprises or hurt feelings.

POST-DELIVERY MEDICATIONS

Pain is subjective. Management of pain is also subjective. The type of birth, the positioning of the baby's head, the length of time you push, the presence of any tearing, and the existence of any hemorrhoids are only some of the wide and varied factors that may determine whether you need medication for pain management after childbirth. In a variety of birth spaces, these medications may be administered during your recovery. There are also a plethora of alternative pain management options to help you cope with discomfort as well.

What follows is a list and descriptions of some common medications you may be prescribed following your birth:

Extra-strength acetaminophen

Tylenol seems to help most with local pain and surgical pain. It decreases inflammation and can help with the discomfort of sore nipples from breastfeeding, surgical pain, and other aches or tenderness.

Ibuprofen

This medication helps with the painful cramping that accompanies the contraction of the uterus down to its pre-pregnant size. Non-steroidal anti-inflammatories such as ibuprofen decrease inflammation. The reduced inflammation, in turn, reduces pain from swelling and tissue trauma on the perineum. These medications also soothe sore muscles and reduce local swelling such as with hemorrhoids.

Percocet or another narcotic

It is exceedingly rare to be prescribed a narcotic following a normal uncomplicated vaginal delivery. Strong narcotics have serious potential for addiction, so their use is reserved for post-operative surgical pain management or other unusual circumstances such as significant perineal lacerations. Narcotics are passed through the breast milk, and parents are also cautioned about the side effects and potential risks when these medications are prescribed.

Stool softener

The first several bowel movements following a vaginal birth will bring on the fear that you will hurt your vagina or perineum, or break stitches. A stool softener does not force you to have a bowel movement but will draw water into the colon to help make your bowel movements softer and more comfortable. It is especially helpful if you have stitches or hemorrhoids. Stool softeners are important for those taking narcotics following a surgical birth because these medications cause constipation, and bearing down with constipation can be uncomfortable to the surgical site.

Laxative

Laxatives are different from stool softeners because they help you move your bowel. Stimulating the bowels is important for those who have had a surgical birth and may be on constipating narcotics.

Your Birth Plan Template

How to Use This Template

Remember that you can use this template as a draft and discussion tool. Use chapters 5 and 6 in this book to cross-reference the areas you are choosing to address. The goal is for you to use the template as a guide while you begin making decisions. Take the time to read through each point, but don't be afraid to skip around the template if you find some decisions easier than others.

As you make some of your initial choices, remember to jot down questions that come up for you to ask your provider, and to determine the specific policies or practices of your chosen birth space. I suggest starting in pencil, leaving room to make changes as you learn more through prenatal education and in discussions with your provider, partner, and designated birth team. I am confident in your ability to make decisions that are right for you and your baby. You are the expert in what works best for you. Your completed birth plan is simply the vehicle you provide to those who care for you. It contains information about you and points specific to your preferences. I hope that through your diligent planning for labor and birth, you experience a birth as magnificent, empowering, and autonomous as can be.

My Preferences for Labor and Birth

These are the preferences to be used to help guide informed decision making along with my care team.

My name and pronouns: _____

You can call me: _____

My due date is: _____

My midwife or physician, or both: _____

Medical information you need to know about me, this pregnancy, or the baby:
(Pregnancy complications, medical diagnoses, or baby gender information can go here.)

_____

_____

_____

My Labor support team includes:

_____ (Title) Contact number _____

_____ (Title) Contact number _____

Important information about my labor support team:

_____

_____

_____

_____

_____

_____

ENVIRONMENT/ATMOSPHERE

☐ Please limit the number of people in my labor space who are not part of my care team.

☐ I would like the lighting to be:
  ☐ Dark
  ☐ Dim
  ☐ Bright

☐ I plan on having music.

☐ I plan on using aromatherapy.

☐ I plan on bringing in the following items from home for comfort or to use as a focal point: _____.

Other important information about the environment:

_____

_____

_____

LABOR PREFERENCES

☐ I plan to defer admission to the labor space until I am in active labor.

☐ I would like to move about freely.

☐ I would like to try many different positions.

☐ I am open to using tools to help with optimal positioning.

☐ I would like to consider alternative methods of starting labor before trying medication.

☐ I prefer not to have an IV. If I need an IV, I would prefer no IV fluids.

Other important information about my labor preferences:
(If you are using a particular pain management strategy such as the Bradley method or HypnoBirthing, it should go here.)

_____

_____

_____

PAIN MANAGEMENT

- ☐ I am aware of my options.
- ☐ I am interested in trying hydrotherapy in a pool, shower, or tub.
- ☐ I would prefer not to use pain medication or an epidural.
- ☐ I plan on using an epidural in active labor.
- ☐ I will consider using IV pain medication.

Other important information about my pain management plan:

(If you prefer not to be offered medications or epidurals, that request should go here.)

_____

_____

_____

SPECIAL TECHNIQUES/MONITORING/CERVICAL EXAMS

- ☐ I prefer the baby be intermittently monitored.
- ☐ If continuous monitoring is necessary, I prefer a portable monitor.
- ☐ I would prefer my amniotic bag to rupture on its own.
- ☐ I would prefer to limit cervical exams, particularly after my water has broken.

_____

_____

_____

BIRTH PREFERENCES

☐ I would like to push in the positions
that feel best for me (squatting, standing,
kneeling, side-lying).

☐ I would like a mirror when my progress gets
close enough to see external progression.

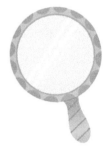

Other information about my birth preferences:

_____

_____

_____

EPISIOTOMY/ASSISTED VAGINAL DELIVERIES/CESAREAN BIRTH

☐ I know that episiotomies and assisted vaginal deliveries are
not routine practice. If these are being considered, I would like
to be advised as soon as possible.

☐ In the event of a cesarean birth:

    ☐ I would like _____ to accompany me to the operating
room with the least amount of separation possible.

    ☐ I would like to see the baby as they are being born.

    ☐ I would prefer delayed cord clamping when possible.

    ☐ I would like _____ to be able to shorten the cord.

    ☐ I would like skin-to-skin contact in the operating room.

    ☐ I would like _____ to perform skin-to-skin
contact in the operating room if I am unable to.

☐ If my baby needs to be separated from me, I
  would like _____ to accompany the baby.

☐ In the event I am separated from my baby,
  I prefer _____ to remain with me.

Other important information about unexpected events during labor:

_____

_____

_____

THIRD STAGE

☐ I would like skin-to-skin contact following the birth.

My plans for the umbilical cord:

☐ Please keep the cord intact. I am planning a lotus birth.

☐ Please allow _____ to cut the cord after it ceases pulsations.

☐ I am planning on cord blood banking.

My plans for the placenta:

☐ I am taking it home with me.

☐ I plan on donating it.

☐ Other _____

Other important information about third stage:

(Preferences for pitocin administration should go here.)

_____

_____

_____

_____

_____

NEWBORN CARE PREFERENCES

☐ I would prefer an uninterrupted first hour of skin-to-skin contact.

☐ I plan on having the following medications administered to my baby this hospitalization:

    ☐ Erythromycin

    ☐ Vitamin K

    ☐ Hepatitis B vaccine

☐ If my baby has a penis, I plan on having my baby circumcised during this hospital stay.

POSTPARTUM RECOVERY PLAN

☐ I plan on _____ remaining with me as I begin my postpartum recovery.

☐ I plan on early discharge if possible.

☐ I plan to breast- or chest-feed exclusively.

☐ I plan on using pumped milk.

☐ I plan on bottle feeding.

☐ I plan on using a combination of feeding methods.

Other information about your postpartum plan:

(Include items such as rooming-in, formula supplementation, and feeding support.)

_____

_____

_____

_____

_____

Other important information:

(Include religious, cultural, or traditional practices, or any specific concerns you have.)

_____

_____

_____

_____

_____

_____

_____

_____

_____

_____

_____

_____

_____

_____

_____

Signatures:

This labor and birth plan have been reviewed by my provider based on my prenatal course.

Healthcare provider signature: _____ DATE: _____

My signature: _____ DATE: _____

References

Akca, Aysu, Aytul Corbacioglu Esmer, Eser Sefik Ozyurek, Arife Aydin, Nazli Korkmaz, Husnu Gorgen, and Ozgur Akbayir. "The Influence of the Systematic Birth Preparation Program on Childbirth Satisfaction." *Archives of Gynecology and Obstetrics* 295, no. 5 (May 2017): 1127–1133. doi: 10.1007/s00404-017-4345-5.

Bieda, Angela, Gerrit Hirschfeld, Pia Schönfeld, Julia Brailovskaia, Muyu Lin, and Jürgen Margraf. "Happiness, Life Satisfaction and Positive Mental Health: Investigating Reciprocal Effects over Four Years in a Chinese Student Sample." *Journal of Research in Personality* 78 (Feb. 2019): 198–209. doi.org/10.1016/j.jrp.2018.11.012.

Blix, Ellen, Robyn Maude, Elisabeth Hals, Sezer Kisa, Elisabeth Karlsen, Ellen Aagaard Nohr, Ank de Jonge, et al. "Intermittent Auscultation Fetal Monitoring during Labour: A Systematic Scoping Review to Identify Methods, Effects, and Accuracy." *PloS One* 14, no. 7 (Jul. 2019): e0219573. doi: 10.1371/journal .pone.0219573.

Brantsaeter, Anne Lise, Margaretha Haugen, Sven Ove Samuelsen, Hanne Torjusen, Lill Trogstad, Jan Alexander, Per Magnus, et al. "A Dietary Pattern Characterized by High Intake of Vegetables, Fruits, and Vegetable Oils Is Associated with Reduced Risk of Preeclampsia in Nulliparous Pregnant Norwegian Women." *Journal of Nutrition* 139, no. 6 (Jun. 2009): 1162–68. doi: 10.3945 /jn.109.104968.

Campbell, Virginia, and Mary Nolan. "'It Definitely Made a Difference': A Grounded Theory Study of Yoga for Pregnancy and Women's Self-efficacy for Labour." *Midwifery* 68 (Jan. 2019): 74–83. doi: 10.1016/j.midw.2018.10.005.

Campolong, Kelsey, Sarah Jenkins, Matthew M. Clark, Kristi Borowski, Nancy Nelson, Katherine M. Moore, and William V.

Bobo. "The Association of Exercise During Pregnancy with Trimester-Specific and Postpartum Quality of Life and Depressive Symptoms in a Cohort of Healthy Pregnant Women." *Archives of Women's Mental Health* 21, no. 2 (Apr. 2018): 215–24. doi: 10.1007/s00737-017-0783-0.

Cheyney, Melissa, Paul Burcher, and Saraswathi Vedam. "A Crusade Against Home Birth." *Birth* 41, no. 1 (March 2014): 1–4. doi: 10.1111/birt.12099.

Coll, Carolina V. N., Marlos Rodrigues Domingues, Alan Stein, Bruna Gonçalves Cordeiro da Silva, Diego G. Bassani, Fernando P. Hartwig, Inácio Crochemore M. da Silva, et al. "Efficacy of Regular Exercise During Pregnancy on the Prevention of Postpartum Depression: The PAMELA Randomized Clinical Trial." *JAMA Network Open* 2, no. 1 (Jan. 2019): e186861. doi: 10.1001/jamanetworkopen.2018.6861.

Dabiri, Fatemeh, and Arefeh Shahi. "The Effect of LI4 Acupressure on Labor Pain Intensity and Duration of Labor: A Randomized Controlled Trial." *Oman Medical Journal* 29, no. 6 (Nov. 2014): 425–29. doi: 10.5001/omj.2014.113.

Danziger, Phoebe, Maria Skoczylas, and Naomi Laventhal. "Parental Refusal of Standard-of-Care Prophylactic Newborn Practices: In One Center's Experience, Many Refuse One But Few Refuse All. *Hospital Pediatrics* 9, no. 6 (Jun. 2019): 429–33. doi: 10.1542/hpeds.2019-0029.

Dayal, Shailja, and Peter L. Hong. "Premature Rupture of Membranes." *StatPearls [Internet]*. Treasure Island, FL: StatPearls Publishing, 2020.

Dekker, Rebecca "Evidence Confirms Birth Centers Provide Top-Notch Care." National Birth Center Study II. American Association of Birth Centers, Jan. 2013. BirthCenters.org/page/nbcsii.

Declercq, Eugene, and Naomi Stotland. "Planned Home Birth." UpToDate. Last modified Aug. 2020. UpToDate.com/contents /planned-home-birth.

De la Chapelle, Arnaud, Michel Carles, V. Gleize, Jean Dellamonica, A. Lallia, Andre Bongain, and Marc Raucoules. "Impact of Walking Epidural Analgesia on Obstetric Outcome of Nulliparous Women in Spontaneous Labour." *International Journal of Obstetric Anesthesia* 15, no. 2 (Apr. 2006): 104–8. doi: 10.1016/j .ijoa.2005.07.002.

Demirel, Gulbahtiyar, and Handan Guler. "The Effect of Uterine and Nipple Stimulation on Induction with Oxytocin and the Labor Process." *Worldviews on Evidence-based Nursing* 12, no. 5 (Oct. 2015): 273–80. doi: 10.1111/wvn.12116.

El-Refaye, Ghada E., Engy M. El Nahas, and Hassan O. Ghareeb. "Effect of Kinesio Taping Therapy Combined with Breathing Exercises on Childbirth Duration and Labor Pain: A Randomized Controlled Trial." *Bulletin of Faculty of Physical Therapy* 21, no. 1 (Aug. 2016): 23–31. doi: 10.4103/1110-6611.188026.

Ferreira, Cátia Liliana Martins, Cláudia Maria Lopes Guerra, Ana Isabel Teixeira Jesus Silva, Helena Rafaela Vieira do Rosário, and Maria Beatriz Ferreira Leite de Oliveira Pereira. "Exercise in Pregnancy: The Impact of an Intervention Program in the Duration of Labor and Mode of Delivery." *Revista Brasileira de Ginecologia e Obstetrícia* 41, no. 2 (Nov. 2018): 68–75. doi: 10.1055/s-0038-1675613.

Garvey, Melissa. The National Birth Center Study II: Research Confirms Low Cesarean Rates and Health Care Costs at Birth Centers. *Midwifery Today with International Midwife* 106 (Summer 2013): 40, 68.

Gbenjo, Joanne, and Elizabeth Leonard. "Does Eating Dates Prior to Labor Hasten Labor Outcomes?" *Evidence-Based Practice* 22, no. 4 (Apr. 2019): 14–15.

Ghaedrahmati, Maryam, Ashraf Kazemi, Gholamreza Kheirabadi, Amrollah Ebrahimi, and Masood Bahrami. "Postpartum Depression Risk Factors: A Narrative Review." *Journal of Education and Health Promotion* 6, no. 60 (Aug. 2017). https://www.ncbi.nlm.nih.gov/pmc/articles/PMC5561681/.

Gomez-Pomar, Enrique, and Robert Blubaugh. "The Baby Friendly Hospital Initiative and the Ten Steps for Successful Breastfeeding: A Critical Review of the Literature." Journal of Perinatology 38, no. 6 (Jun. 2018): 623–32. doi: 10.1038/s41372-018-0068-0.

Gourounti, Kleanthi, and Jane Sandall. "Admission Cardiotocography Versus Intermittent Auscultation of Fetal Heart Rate: Effects on Neonatal Apgar Score, on the Rate of Caesarean Sections and on the Rate of Instrumental Delivery—A Systematic Review." *International Journal of Nursing Studies* 44, no. 6 (Aug. 2007): 1029–35. doi: 10.1016/j.ijnurstu.2006.06.002.

Hellams, Audrey, Taylor Sprague, Christina Saldanha, and Mark Archambault. "Nitrous Oxide for Labor Analgesia." *Journal of the American Academy of Physician Assistants* 31, no. 1 (Jan. 2018): 41–44. doi: 10.1097/01.JAA.0000527700.00698.8c.

Ignatov, Tanja, Holm Eggemann, Serban Dan Costa, and Atanas Ignatov. "Perinatal and Maternal Outcomes at Term in Low-Risk Pregnancies According to NICE Criteria: Comparison Between a Tertiary Obstetrical Hospital and Midwife-Attended Units." *Archives of Gynecology and Obstetrics* 296, no. 2 (Jun. 2017): 223–29. doi: 10.1007/s00404-017-4423-8.

Jhala, Akshaykumari. "A Study to Assess the Effectiveness of Lamaze Breathing on Labor Pain and Anxiety Towards Labor Outcome among Primigravida Mothers During Labor in Community Health Center, Kolar Road, Bhopal." Indian Journal of Obstetrics and Gynecology 5, no. 1 (Jan.–Mar. 2017): 19–22. doi: 10.21088/ijog.2321.1636.5117.2.

Kahalon, Rotem, Heidi Preis, and Yael Benyamini. "Who Benefits Most from Skin-to-Skin Mother-Infant Contact After Birth? Survey Findings on Skin-To-Skin and Birth Satisfaction by Mode of Birth." *Midwifery* 92 (Oct. 2020). https://www.science -direct.com/science/article/abs/pii/S0266613820302345.

Laelago, Tariku. "Herbal Medicine Use During Pregnancy: Benefits and Untoward Effects." In *Herbal Medicine*, by Philip F. Builders. Accessed *IntechOpen* (Nov. 2018). doi: 10.5772 /intechopen.76896.

Louis-Jacques, Adetola, and Alison Stuebe. "Long-term Maternal Benefits of Breastfeeding: Longer Durations of Breastfeeding Are Associated with Improved Health Outcomes for Mothers and Should Be Supported by Ob/Gyns." *Contemporary Ob/Gyn* 63, no. 7 (Jul. 2018): 26-29.

Martis, Ruth, Ova Emilia, Detty S. Nurdiati, and Julie Brown. "Intermittent Auscultation (IA) of Fetal Heart Rate in Labour for Fetal WellBeing." *Cochrane Database of Systematic Reviews* 2, no. 2 (Feb. 2017): CD008680. doi: 10.1002/14651858.CD008680.pub2.

McRae, Maureen J. "Exclusive Breastfeeding, 24-Hour Rooming-In, and the Importance of Women's Informed Choices." *Nursing for Women's Health* 23, no. 4 (Jul. 2019): 309–15. doi: 10.1016/j .nwh.2019.05.003.

Moore, Mary Lou. "Breastfeeding Benefits Support–Research." *Scientific Journal of Gynecology and Obstetrics* 1, no. 1 (2018): 001–002.

Munn, Allison C., Susan D. Newman, Martina Mueller, Shannon M. Phillips, and Sarah N. Taylor. "The Impact in the United States of the Baby-Friendly Hospital Initiative on Early Infant Health and Breastfeeding Outcomes." *Breastfeeding Medicine* 11, no. 5 (Jun. 2016): 222–30. doi: 10.1089/bfm.2015.0135.

Ng, Chin Ang, Jacqueline J. Ho, and Zcho Huey Lee. "The Effect of Rooming-in on Duration of Breastfeeding: A Systematic Review of Randomised and Non-randomised Prospective Controlled Studies." *PloS One* 14, no. 4 (Apr. 2019): e0215869. doi: 10.1371/journal.pone.0215869.

Papandreou, Christopher, Nerea Becerra-Tomás, Mònica Bulló, Miguel Ángel Martínez-González, Dolores Corella, Ramon Estruch, Emilio Ros, et al. "Legume Consumption and Risk of All-Cause, Cardiovascular, and Cancer Mortality in the PREDIMED Study." *Clinical Nutrition* 38, no. 1 (Feb. 2019): 348–56. doi: 10.1016/j.clnu.2017.12.019.

Preston, Roanne. "Walking Epidurals for Labour Analgesia: Do They Benefit Anyone?" *Canadian Journal of Anesthesia* 57, no. 2 (Feb. 2010): 103–6. doi: 10.1007/s12630-009-9229-0.

Puia, Denise. "First-Time Mothers' Experiences of a Planned Cesarean Birth." *The Journal of Perinatal Education* 27, no. 1 (2018): 50–60. doi: 10.1891/1058-1243.27.1.50.

Qumer, Shahnaj, and Debalina Ghosh. (2019). "Effectiveness of Patterned Breathing Technique on Pain During First Stage of Labour-A Narrative Review." *International Journal of Nursing Education* 11, no. 3 (2019): 60. https://www.researchgate.net/publication/334417756_Effectiveness_of_Patterned_Breathing_Technique_on_Pain_During_First_Stage_of_Labour-A_Narrative_Review.

Rahimi, Farzneh, Shadi Goli, Nages Soltani, Habibolah Rezaei, and Zahra Amouzeshi. "Effects of Complementary Therapies on Labor Pain: A Literature Review." *Modern Care Journal* 15, no. 1 (2018): https://www.researchgate.net/publication/325117764_Effects_of_Complementary_Therapies_on_Labor_Pain_A_Literature_Review.

Rungruangmaitree, Runchana, and Wannee Jiraungkoorskul. "Pea, *Pisum sativum*, and Its Anticancer Activity." *Pharmacognosy Review* 11, no. 21 (Jan.–Jun. 2017): 39–42. doi: 10.4103/phrev .phrev_57_16.

Sánchez-Chino, Xariss, Cristian Jiménez-Martínez, Gloria Dávila-Ortiz, Isela Álvarez-González, and Eduardo Madrigal-Bujaidar. "Nutrient and Nonnutrient Components of Legumes, and Its Chemopreventive Activity: A Review." *Nutrition and Cancer* 67, no. 3 (Feb. 2015): 401–10. doi: 10.1080/01635581.2015.1004729.

Schlaeger, Judith M., Elizabeth M. Gabzdyl, Jeanie L. Bussell, Nobuari Takakura, Hiroyoshi Yajima, Miho Takayama, and Diana J. Wilkie. "Acupuncture and Acupressure in Labor." *Journal of Midwifery and Women's Health* 62, no. 1 (Dec. 2016): 12–28. doi: 10.1111/jmwh.12545.

Stapleton, Susan Rutledge, Cara Osborne, Jessica Illuzzi. "Outcomes of Care in Birth Centers: Demonstration of a Durable Model." *Journal of Midwifery and Women's Health* 58, no. 1 (Jan./Feb. 2013): 3–14. https://pubmed.ncbi.nlm.nih.gov/23363029/.

Steptoe, Andrew. "Happiness and Health." *Annual Review of Public Health* 40 (Apr. 2019): 339–59. doi: 10.1146 /annurev-publhealth-040218-044150.

Tasseau, A., Elizabeth Walter-Nicolet, and F. Autre. "Management of Healthy Newborns in the Delivery Room and Maternal Satisfaction." *Archives de Pédiatrie* 25, no. 5 (Jun. 2018): 309–14. doi: 10.1016/j.arcped.2018.05.010.

Thuvarakan, Kenoja, Henrik Zimmermann, Morten Kold Mikkelsen, and Parisa Gazerani. "Transcutaneous Electrical Nerve Stimulation as a Pain-Relieving Approach in Labor Pain: A Systematic Review and MetaAnalysis of Randomized Controlled

Trials." *Neuromodulation: Technology at the Neural Interface* 23, no. 6 (Jul. 2020): 732–46. doi: 10.1111/ner.13221.

U.S. Prevention Services Task Force, Curry, Susan J., Alex H. Krist, Douglas K. Owens, Michael J. Barry, Aaron B. Caughey, Karina W. Davidson, et al. "Ocular Prophylaxis for Gonococcal Ophthalmia Neonatorum: US Preventive Services Task Force Reaffirmation Recommendation Statement." *The Journal of the American Medical Association* 321, no. 4 (Jan. 2019): 394–98. doi: 10.1001/jama.2018.21443.

Wadhwa, Yogyata, Ahmad H. Alghadir, and Zaheen A. Iqbal. "Effect of Antenatal Exercises, Including Yoga, on the Course of Labor, Delivery and Pregnancy: A Retrospective Study." *International Journal of Environmental Research and Public Health* 17, no. 15 (Jul. 2020): 5274. doi: 10.3390/ijerph17155274.

Werner, Elizabeth, Maia Miller, Lauren M. Osborne, Sierra Kuzava, and Catherine Monk. "Preventing Postpartum Depression: Review and Recommendations." *Archives of Women's Mental Health* 18, no. 1 (Feb. 2015): 41–60. doi: 10.1007/s00737-014-0475-y.

Zamawe, Collins, Carina King, Hannah Maria Jennings, Chrispin Mandiwa, and Edward Fottrell. "Effectiveness and Safety of Herbal Medicines for Induction of Labour: A Systematic Review and Meta-Analysis." *BMJ Open* 8, no. 10 (Oct. 2018): e022499. doi: 10.1136/bmjopen-2018-022499.

Index

Acknowledgments

To Jamie, who has remained certain of my successes even when I was unable to see the finish line. To Jasmyn, Jaymie, Jayar, and Jesse, who allowed my body to be the vessel from which they arrived, which will never not blow my mind. I love you all ferociously. To my patients, who have trusted their bodies and their babies to my care, there will be no greater honor than to continue to care for you. To the grand midwives, who initiated and carried the tradition of caring for the African-American community of birthers well before birth was moved from our homes. In your honor, I will not forget that respectful birth is our human right, and I will continue to fight for this justice in your honor. To those at Callisto who trusted me to create this work using terms that convey my reverence to all humans who grow humans.

About the Author

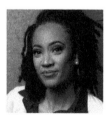

Dr. **Stephanie Mitchell** is a certified nurse midwife. She developed the "Intermittent Auscultation Checklist," which helps labor and delivery providers of medical industrial complexes identify candidates for low-intervention labor and birth. Dr. Mitchell is building Birth Sanctuary Gainesville, which will be the first free-standing birth center in the state to serve the rural and surrounding birthing communities. Connect with her on Instagram @Doctor_Midwife.

T

Tea, red raspberry leaf, 16

TENS units, 111

Tranquilizers, 108

U

Umbilical cord cutting, 28, 119

V

Vaccines, 124–125

Vacuum-assisted deliveries, 116

Vaginal birth after a cesarean
(VBAC), 118

Visitors, 129

Visualizations, 8, 9–10

Vitamin K, 32–33, 124

Vocalizations, 109

W

Walking
as exercise, 18
to induce labor, 102

Water breaking, 23, 101

Y

Yoga, 18

Acknowledgments

To Jamie, who has remained certain of my successes even when I was unable to see the finish line. To Jasmyn, Jaymie, Jayar, and Jesse, who allowed my body to be the vessel from which they arrived, which will never not blow my mind. I love you all ferociously. To my patients, who have trusted their bodies and their babies to my care, there will be no greater honor than to continue to care for you. To the grand midwives, who initiated and carried the tradition of caring for the African-American community of birthers well before birth was moved from our homes. In your honor, I will not forget that respectful birth is our human right, and I will continue to fight for this justice in your honor. To those at Callisto who trusted me to create this work using terms that convey my reverence to all humans who grow humans.

About the Author

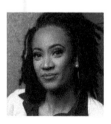 Dr. **Stephanie Mitchell** is a certified nurse midwife. She developed the "Intermittent Auscultation Checklist," which helps labor and delivery providers of medical industrial complexes identify candidates for low-intervention labor and birth. Dr. Mitchell is building Birth Sanctuary Gainesville, which will be the first free-standing birth center in the state to serve the rural and surrounding birthing communities. Connect with her on Instagram @Doctor_Midwife.